ANCIENT
GRAINS

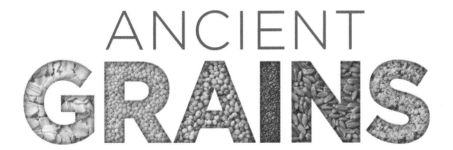

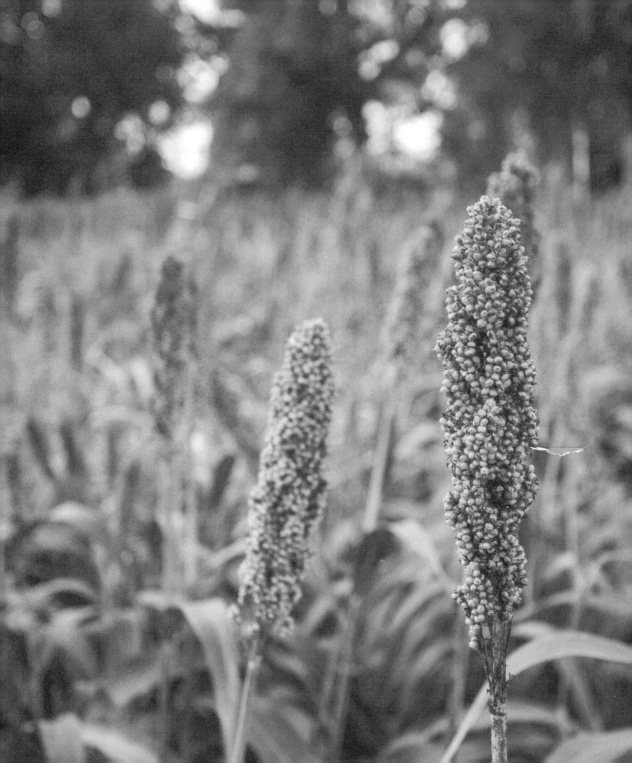

ANCIENT
GRAINS

A Guide to Cooking with Power-Packed
Millet, Oats, Spelt, Farro, Sorghum & Teff

KIM LUTZ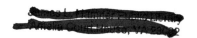

FOREWORD BY STEPHANIE PEDERSEN

STERLING
New York

STERLING
New York

An Imprint of Sterling Publishing Co., Inc.
1166 Avenue of the Americas
New York, NY 10036

ISBN 978-1-4549-1937-7

Distributed in Canada by Sterling Publishing Co., Inc.
c/o Canadian Manda Group, 664 Annette Street
Toronto, Ontario, Canada M6S 2C8
Distributed in the United Kingdom by GMC Distribution Services
Castle Place, 166 High Street, Lewes, East Sussex, England BN7 1XU
Distributed in Australia by Capricorn Link (Australia) Pty. Ltd.
P.O. Box 704, Windsor, NSW 2756, Australia

For information about custom editions, special sales, and premium and corporate purchases,
please contact Sterling Special Sales at 800-805-5489 or specialsales@sterlingpublishing.com.

Manufactured in Canada

2 4 6 8 10 9 7 5 3 1

www.sterlingpublishing.com

Image Credits

All photography by Bill Milne Photography, except: Alamy: © Steffen Hauser/botanikfoto: ix, © WILDLIFE GmbH:
104; Depositphotos: © Kris Cole: 101, © Givaga: 57, © Anton Ignatenco: 88, © Masayoshi Kusai: 94, © mvw@tut.by: 68,
© photomaru: 55, © rozmarina: 93, © rrraum: 20, © scis65: 23, © Marek Uliasz: 11, © Joanna Wnuk: 5; Getty
Images: © Julio Etchart/Robert Harding World Imagery: xvi, © Kevin Law/All Canada Photos: xi; iStockphoto:
© duckycards: 50, © WiktorD: 61; Shutterstock: © AnastasiiaM: 14, © Chailalla: ii, © DronG: 32, © Brent Hofacker:
13, © Ekaterina Kondratova: 2, © Jerry Lin: xii, © Maks Narodenko: 35, 65, © olvius: xiv, © Harald Walker: 9, © Jeff
Wasserman: 7, © Mahathir Mohd Yasin: vi, © Suthiphong Yina: xvii

For Steve, Casey, and Evan.

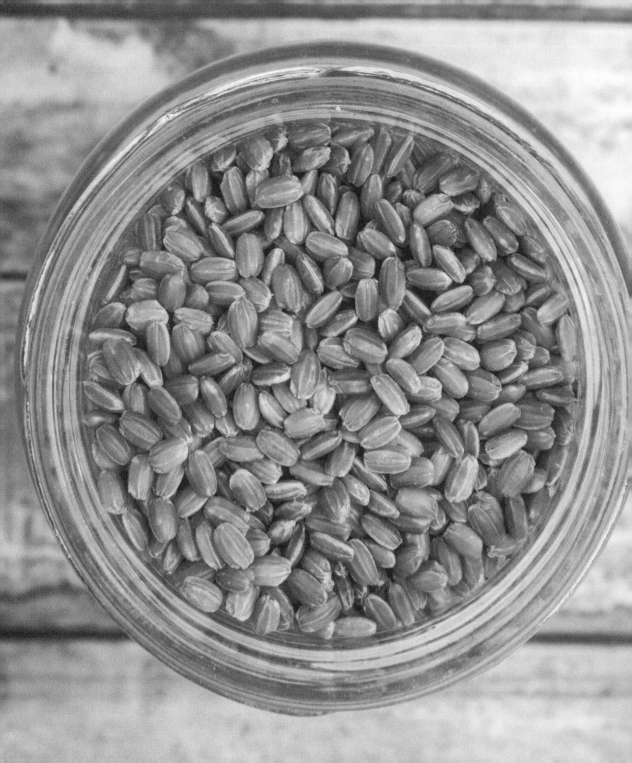

CONTENTS

If you look back into your family's culinary history, you'll probably find many well-loved recipes based on grains. In the introduction to this book, Kim Lutz shares her memories of the delicious loaves of millet bread her aunts made as a special treat. In my family, oats were ingredients that my Danish grandmother always enjoyed and made into a comforting porridge. One of my close friends, whose family hails from Italy, loves farro—and another dear friend, whose family is German, has a way with spelt.

When our children become adults and look back on their formative years, what grain, other than wheat, will they remember? I ask because for the last fifty years or so, wheat has been the most heavily used grain—at least in North America. But change is in the air. An increasing number of health experts are now decrying the dangers of eating wheat and processed grains, linking them to diabetes, cancer, autoimmune disease, and obesity, a point of view that has been taken up by the authors of books with titles like *Wheat Belly: Lose the Wheat, Lose the Weight, and Find Your Path Back to Health* and *Grain Brain: The Surprising Truth about Wheat, Carbs, and Sugar—Your Brain's Silent Killers*, as well as the proponents of popular diets, from Atkins to Paleo. Now that wheat and processed grains have such a bad reputation in these influential circles, I can't help but wonder: What's to become of the grains that have fed and nourished humans since the beginning of time?

Happily, you'll soon discover that the future of ancient grains, such as farro, spelt, millet, oats, sorghum, and teff is assured. Thanks to Kim Lutz, you'll see how easy (and delicious) it is to replace processed wheat and simple carbs with healthy whole grains.

You'll get all the details about the nutritional value and culinary possibilities of these ancient grains for every meal of the day (including desserts) in Kim's brilliant book, but here's a quick sketch of each—just enough information, I hope, to whet your interest—and your appetite.

FARRO

This ancient whole-wheat grain fed most of the Mediterranean for centuries, including the Roman Empire. The nutty taste and toothsome texture of this popular cooking grain have won the hearts of foodies, who love to eat it in salads, as a replacement for rice in risotto, as a quick side dish, or tossed into the soup pot to add extra texture,

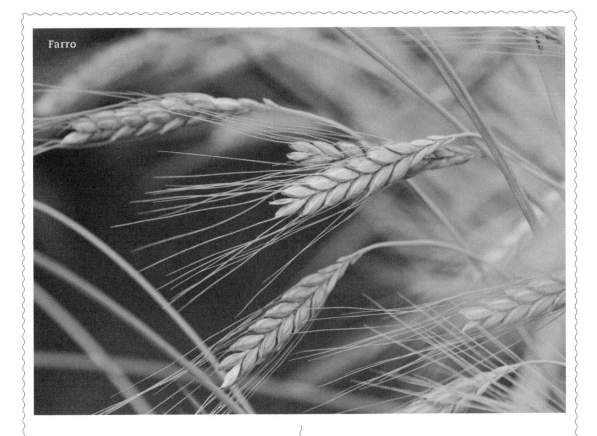

Farro

flavor, and nutrition. Or do what I do: Toss a quarter of a cup of cooked farro into your favorite bran muffin or oatmeal cookie recipe. Nutritionists love the grain's high fiber content, protein, iron, magnesium, and zinc, as well as lignans—phytonutrients that are high in antioxidants. A word about lignans: In a study of lignans and endometrial cancer performed by researchers from Northern California Cancer Institute in Union City, California, and published in the August 2003 issue of *Journal of the National Cancer Institute*, 500 women between the age of 25 and 79 were studied. The women with the highest intakes of plant lignans had the lowest risk of endometrial cancer.

SPELT

Much like farro, spelt can be ground into a flour or used as a cooking grain. A staple food in pre-Medieval Europe, spelt's generous levels of protein, fiber, niacin, thiamine, iron, magnesium, manganese, phosphorus, and zinc make it an important addition to modern meals, as well. Spelt is high in dietary fiber and may play an important role in managing type 2 diabetes and preventing heart disease. According to a twelve-week study of 233 people, featured in the October 2010 issue of *The American Journal of Clinical Nutrition*, eating three servings of whole grains daily can significantly reduce cardiovascular disease risk in middle-aged people by lowering blood pressure. Kim has some great suggestions for using spelt, including my favorite, the brilliant Hummus Arugula Flatbread!

MILLET

A small-seeded grass that grows in hot, dry climates, millet is perhaps best known these days as birdseed, but it has a long and vaunted history as one of the world's oldest and best-loved grains. Indeed, millet is referenced in ancient Chinese texts, as well as the Bible. This supergrain is a rich source of fiber, protein, magnesium, manganese, phosphorus, and copper, as well as phytonutrients such as lignans. I love to stir a bit of cooked millet into pancake, waffle, and muffin batters, and it's fantastic cooked with coconut milk as a breakfast porridge. A three-year study of 229 postmenopausal women with heart disease, published in the July 2005 issue of *American Heart Journal*, showed that women who ate at least six servings of whole grains (including millet) each week, experienced slowed progression of atherosclerosis, the build-up of plaque that narrows blood vessels.

OATS

The ultimate comfort food, oats are one of the most popular whole grains in North America (after wheat). Oats are inexpensive and easily found in supermarkets everywhere, but best of all, they are a nutritional powerhouse, with generous supplies of manganese, molybdenum, phosphorus, copper, biotin, vitamin B1, magnesium, fiber, chromium, zinc, and protein. When they're cooked, rolled or steel-cut oats make a hearty breakfast cereal—and who doesn't love oatmeal cookies and muffins? Groats (whole, hulled oats) are also delicious in salads, pilafs, and sautés of all kinds. No matter how you enjoy oats, aim to have them weekly; the fiber in oats is soluble, and a range of studies over the last two decades has shown that oat consumption is associated with reductions in LDL cholesterol levels. In addition, a study performed by researchers at Sichuan University, China, and published in the December 2015 issue of *Nutrients*, found that oat consumption also lowered blood sugar levels in individuals with type 2 diabetes.

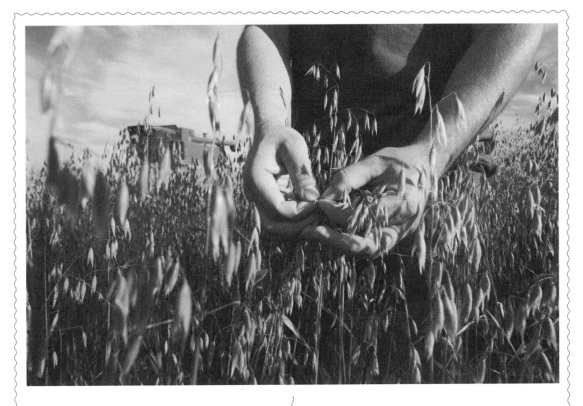

SORGHUM

A favorite among gluten-free bakers, sorghum flour lends a winning tenderness to wheat-free baked goods. But sorghum is so much more versatile than wheat! This small grain, prepared throughout Africa as a porridge or flatbread, can also be made into a couscous-like side dish—the perfect addition to curries and stews. (Sorghum is even used industrially as ethanol.) This hardworking ancient grain contains riboflavin, thiamine, niacin, magnesium, iron, copper, calcium, phosphorus, and—as you'll learn from Kim—large amounts of protein and fiber. Sorghum has been studied for its role in lowering cancer risk, blood sugar, and even cholesterol levels. In a study published in the September 2005 issue of *Journal of Nutrition*, scientists from the University of Nebraska fed different levels of sorghum lipids to hamsters for four weeks, and found that the healthy fats in sorghum significantly reduced bad (LDL) cholesterol . Reductions ranged from 18 percent, in hamsters that were fed a diet that included 0.5 percent sorghum lipids, to 69 percent, in hamsters that were fed a diet that included 5 percent sorghum lipids. Good (HDL) cholesterol was not affected. Researchers concluded that "grain sorghum contains beneficial components that could be used as food ingredients or dietary supplements to manage cholesterol levels in humans."

TEFF

This teensy-weensy grain—native to Eritrea and Ethiopia—measures just one thirty-secondth of an inch in diameter. It takes 3,000 grains of teff to make up one gram. But despite its diminutive size, teff is a nutritional giant, boasting protein, fiber, iron, magnesium, and more calcium than any other grain. Teff also contains vitamin B6 and vitamin C. Believed to be one of the world's first domesticated crops, teff has fed people since at least the time of the pharaohs. Its culinary uses are many: Teff can be made into a porridge or mixed with water and fermented and cooked into the Ethiopian flatbread, injera; it is a popular ingredient in veggie burgers; and it is becoming more and more commonly used as a gluten-free flour in a raft of applications. However, teff is just now earning a place in the halls of scientific research. In fact, one study on celiac disease by researchers at Leiden University Medical Center in the Netherlands, and published in the October 2005 issue of

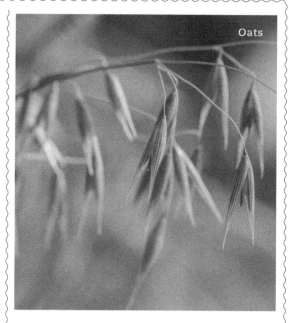

Oats

New England Journal of Medicine, found teff to be a safe, nutritious, gluten-free stand-in for wheat flour.

GET STARTED WITH ANCIENT GRAINS

If you've never cooked with any of these amazing grains, choose one and explore! Let *Ancient Grains* be your guidebook. Kim Lutz is committed to developing recipes for delicious food that will strengthen your body, enhance your health, and boost your energy. She is also committed to making it accessible. I have watched Kim give recipe demonstrations: She is always down-to-earth, real, and generous in sharing her own experience.

Like you, Kim has a lot going on: She's a mother, wife, food expert, author, and an active member of her community. She's busy and she knows that you're busy. Kim gets that you're probably not spending hours in the kitchen, dehydrating and soaking and pulverizing and mincing. The recipes in this book are designed to make adding ancients grains to your life easy and fun. First off, Kim walks you through purchasing and storing grains, so you get the most for your money. Next, she offers great information on cook-ahead grains that can be refrigerated and used throughout the week in a variety of dishes, or frozen as a do-it-yourself convenience food for use a month later. (Just imagine how easy dinnertime could be with a stash of precooked grains, ready to grab and use!) You'll learn how to cook grains in the slow cooker, on the stovetop, in the oven, and even in the microwave.

As much as we love healthy recipes that are easy and speedy to make, we also want our grains to taste good, too, right? So good that we won't go running back to white bread, white rice, or instant oatmeal anytime soon. Fortunately, the recipes in *Ancient Grains* are scrumptious! Some of my personal favorites are: Creamy Sunrise Smoothie (it's more like a milkshake—only so much more nourishing—thanks to ingredients like oats, fruit, carrots, and hemp), Nutty Granola (this is a great no-sugar version), and toothsome Mushroom Sorghum Soup (a delicious way to experiment with sorghum). In addition to these recipes, you'll also find a generous array of breakfast foods, lunch dishes, drinks, snacks, dinner entrees, and desserts, so you'll have no trouble finding plenty of new favorites to suit your taste. Whether you are vegan, avoiding gluten, prefer not to use mainstream sweeteners, or have other dietary concerns, Kim keeps your needs in mind. The recipes in *Ancient Grains* are eminently flexible, with adaptations for a wide range of preferences.

More than 75 recipes and pages and pages of great information are ahead—just turn the page to get started! Knowing how to use and enjoy ancient grains is going to change the way you and your loved ones eat—for the better.

To your health!

Much love,
Stephanie Pedersen

Author of *Berries: The Complete Guide to Cooking with Power-Packed Berries* (Sterling); *Coconut: The Complete Guide to the World's Most Versatile Superfood* (Sterling); *Kale: The Complete Guide to the World's Most Powerful Superfood* (Sterling); and coauthor (with Wayne Coates, PhD) of *Chia: The Complete Guide to the Ultimate Superfood* (Sterling)

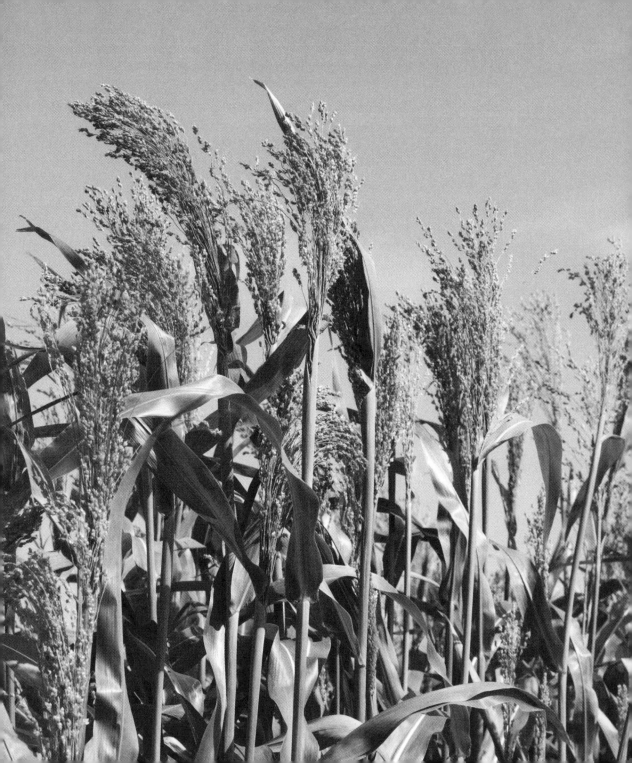

My aunts Ellyn and Nancy gave me my first taste of ancient grains. They are terrific bakers and one of their specialties is millet bread. The warm, crusty loaves dotted with crunchy yellow balls of millet were a special treat. As I was growing up, this delicious bread was the only way I knew to enjoy an ancient grain.

Years later, I am faced with the modern conundrum of trying to eat healthfully in the midst of a very busy schedule. Food companies make it all too easy to grab a toaster pastry for breakfast, chow down on a packaged lunch box, or pop a frozen meal into the microwave for dinner. This ease can be alluring, especially when I'm looking at a day that is jam-packed before I even get out of bed: between work, running to the grocery store, shuttling the kids to sports practice, and doing a couple of loads of laundry, there's little space for thinking about what to serve for dinner—all of which makes the idea of using processed foods very enticing. But the convenience of these foods comes with a cost. The companies that make processed foods use a load of unwholesome ingredients—a lot of white sugar, salt, white flour, and bad-quality fats—to achieve textures and flavors that are appealing. Nutrition is added artificially, via supplements, instead of using fresh, whole foods that are full of real nutrients.

My aunts know what they're doing. Power-packed ancient grains—millet, oats, spelt, farro, sorghum, and teff—make it much easier to eat healthfully naturally. These grains are a pleasure to use, they're loaded with nutrients, and—best of all—they taste delicious.

With a kitchen stocked with ancient grains, I'm far less vulnerable to the siren song of colorful packaging and promises of instant gratification. With little effort, I can prepare a jar of Basic Overnight Oats (page 30) for a breakfast that will fuel me with complex carbohydrates, protein, fiber, and iron. The fiber in this simple meal will keep me from feeling hungry until lunchtime, and the complex carbohydrates will provide the slow-burning energy I need to keep me going as I accomplish my to-do list.

If you're pondering what to have for lunch, Millet Tabbouleh (page 51) is loaded with fresh vegetables and herbs and is just the kind of satisfying lunch that can be prepared and eaten quickly. Crunchy cucumbers, juicy tomatoes, and stick-to-your ribs millet make for a nutrient-rich salad that will please your taste buds as it powers you through the day. The manganese in millet will also contribute to healthy bones and skin.

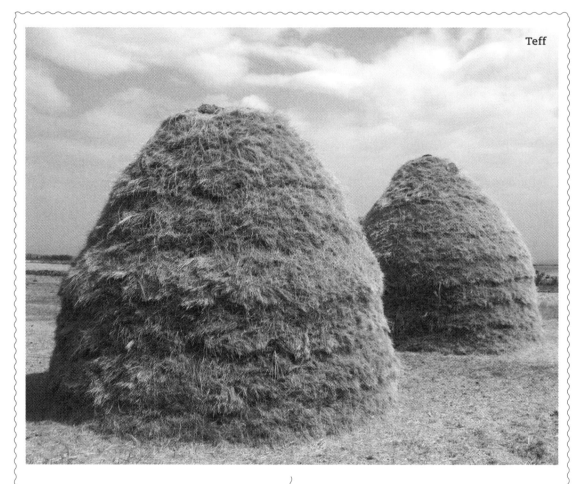

Teff

Coming home at the end of the day and preparing a low-fat, protein-rich Mushroom Sorghum Soup (page 44) and whole-grain Spelt Sandwich Loaf (page 73) won't keep you in the kitchen for long and will end your day in the most delicious way. The phosphorus and iron in sorghum will keep your blood and bones healthy and strong, too.

You'll discover that ancient grains are flexible players in the kitchen. I can transform them in multiple ways to create a wide range of nourishing dishes. For example, I grind sorghum in a nut and seed grinder (or in a clean coffee grinder) to make my own flour, which I can then add to other flours to make protein-rich, gluten-free flour blends that offer deep and nourishing flavors and textures.

In this book you'll learn not only how to make your own nutritious flours for bread and other baked goods, you'll also discover how to blend rolled oats with water in order to make a delicious nondairy milk that can be used in your coffee, served with Nutty Granola (page 39), and stirred into countless recipes. Using this technique, you'll have fresh nondairy milk in minutes, if you've soaked the oats earlier, and you can make only the amount you need.

But that's not all. You can make your own homemade pasta with whole-grain spelt flour in about the same amount of time it takes to boil a big pot of water. After dinner you can enjoy all the health benefits of whole-grain spelt flour in a slice of Blueberry Pie with Whole-Grain Crust (page 101).

You'll soon discover how easy it is to use ancient grains in myriad ways. For example, if you keep a batch of prepared millet, sorghum, or teff in your refrigerator or freezer, you can quickly create filling salads, soups, and entrées. The temptation to grab a lackluster, overprocessed frozen meal quickly evaporates when you have the option to pull together a flavor-filled, hearty Salsa Millet Hash (page 34) instead.

Grains such as millet, sorghum, spelt, farro, teff, and oats have sustained people across Asia, Africa, Europe, and the Americas for thousands of years. Now these ancient

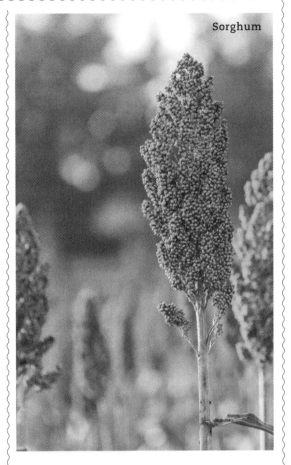

Sorghum

grains are enjoying a resurgence in popularity as superfoods, and for good reason: they supply a powerhouse of nutrition that can easily be parlayed into a wide range of dishes and menus that fit readily into our busy lives and keep us feeling healthy and well fed. Read on to learn how to make these versatile, ancient grains part of your diet every day, and at every meal.

—Kim Lutz

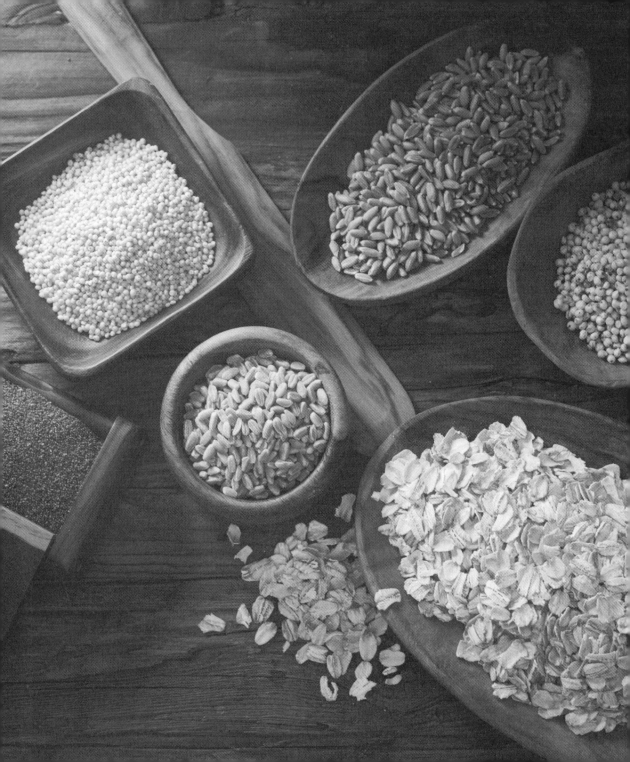

CHAPTER 1

GETTING TO KNOW ANCIENT GRAINS

Ancient grains have remained relatively the same over hundreds and even thousands of years: millet, farro, spelt, sorghum, teff, and oats have not been altered significantly through breeding and hybridization efforts and therefore are very similar to the grains that have been enjoyed by people throughout time. In fact, grains have been an important part of the human diet since the beginning of time, when grasses grew wild and early hunter-gatherers ate them along with other foods that were available to them.

Not all grains are equal within the context of improving our health and nutrition. When we refer to a "grain," what we're really talking about is the seed or kernel of a cereal crop—a type of grass. There is evidence of early Homo sapiens collecting, processing, and eating grains like sorghum 100,000 years ago. An article published by ScienceDaily.com in 2009 reported that archeologists had unearthed evidence that modern humans used wild grains and tubers as far back as the Stone Age. And yet, while grains have been enjoyed for thousands of years all across the globe, different grains are prevalent in different parts of the world. This variety is due to climate, tradition, and availability.

Modern farming and food distribution have created a scenario where the high yields and ease of processing certain grains have allowed them to overtake the market. In an effort to feed as many people as possible during the Green Revolution after World War II (a time of increased technology and initiatives to increase crop yields), a lot of energy went into creating wheat plants that would have high yields and be easy to harvest. These new wheat plants were the result of purposeful hybridization efforts. A lot of good came from these efforts, as more food was available to hungry people across the planet. The spread of this easy-to-grow wheat, however, meant that other grains were neglected and simply not considered for consumer use.

Recently, however, that scenario has started to change. Everything that's old is new again when you're talking about grains.

For one thing, people are learning about the many health benefits of eating whole grains along with lots of fresh fruits and vegetables. Grains such as millet, sorghum, spelt, farro, teff, and oats provide a wide range of nutrients that can help us look and feel our best.

Ancient grains can also be helpful for people who need to follow special diets for health reasons or lifestyle choices. For example, oats, sorghum, millet, and teff can broaden the menu for people who can't eat gluten, due to celiac disease or gluten intolerance. And all of these grains can broaden the food choices available to those who follow a vegetarian or vegan diet.

AN INTRODUCTION TO ANCIENT GRAINS

In order to know how to use ancient grains and incorporate them into your diet, you have to get to know them first—what they look like, where they grow, in what forms they are available, and how to store them.

MILLET

"Millet" refers to a group of plants—indigenous grasses that are grown as a crop in many parts of the world—that produce a small, hard seed. These seeds are usually yellow or beige in color and relatively round.

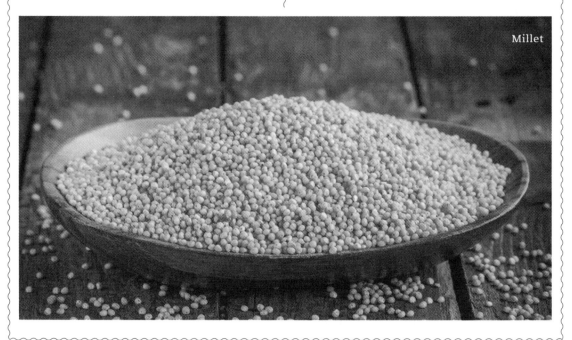

Millet

Millet seeds have inedible hulls that must be removed before the millet can be eaten. There are a few varieties that make up most of the millet grown around the world: Pearl, Foxtail, Proso, and Finger. Because it grows well in hot, dry climates, millet is grown in Africa, South Asia (including India), and the southern United States. It is believed that millet was first enjoyed in Asia over 10,000 years ago, and then made its way across the Black Sea into southern Europe and then into Africa. Because millet can withstand harsh growing conditions, its popularity is on the rise. It can play an important role in feeding people, particularly in drought-ridden places.

Millet is grown as a food crop as well as for hay to feed farm animals and wildlife. In the United States, millet is easily recognizable, because it is the primary component of many commercial types of birdseed. One of the advantages of growing it in your garden, if you have enough space and live in a warm, dry climate (like in Texas), is that it will provide welcome cover to many different kinds of birds and wildlife. A good rule of thumb is if you have the space and ability to grow corn, you can probably grow millet, too.

Millet is becoming increasingly available in the grocery store, both in packages and in the bulk aisle of well-stocked supermarkets.

WHAT'S THE DIFFERENCE BETWEEN GRAINS AND SEEDS?

With more and more interest in healthy eating and incorporating whole foods in our diets, whole grains have received a lot of attention. Not all whole "grains," however, are actually grains—they're seeds. If you're confused (understandably!) about which is which, a basic rule of thumb is: grains are the whole seeds of cereal grasses, like wheat, spelt, farro (also known as emmer), sorghum, millet, teff, rye, barley, and rice. Seeds, on the other hand, come from broadleaf plants, not cereal grasses. In today's natural food marketplace, seeds like amaranth and quinoa are often lumped together with grains (and marketed as grains), but, again, amaranth and quinoa are seeds because they come from broadleaf plants, not cereal grasses. To learn more about the health benefits and culinary uses of seeds, check out my book *Super Seeds* (Sterling 2014), which is loaded with easy, nutritious, delicious recipes that use these tiny, power-packed foods.

Although many mass-market convenience foods are filled with unhealthy ingredients, there are some high-quality options that feature healthier ingredients available, too. If you're looking for prepared foods that contain the whole grain, you can enjoy puffed millet cereal, multigrain crackers and breads that contain millet, and even multigrain tortilla chips.

Incorporating millet into your cooking can be fairly seamless. Millet cooks up fluffy like rice and can take its place in stir-fries, soups, and entrées. Millet is gluten-free, so it can bring nutrition and diversity to meals for anyone who needs to avoid the gluten in wheat, rye, and barley. Millet Porridge (page 30), Millet Tabbouleh (page 51), and Potato Millet Croquettes (page 58) highlight the range of uses that this versatile grain can bring to any diet plan.

Millet, like any grain, can become rancid if it is not stored properly. I like to buy a few pounds of millet at a time. This gives me enough to use when I need it, but not so much that it will go bad before I use it up. The price for a 28-ounce bag of millet is comparable to the cost of a similar-size bag of good-quality brown rice. Millet will last longer if it's kept cold, so I store mine in the refrigerator. If I know that I'm not going to finish it in two or three weeks, I move it to the freezer, where it can stay fresh for at least three to four months.

I also like to batch-cook millet so that I can easily throw together a meal. I cook millet in water (see instructions on page 24), then store it in two-cup amounts in freezer-safe containers. I keep at least one of these in the refrigerator so that I can use it throughout the week. The rest I put in the freezer, so that I can add a whole-grain boost to soups, stews, or salads as I make them over the next three to four months.

SORGHUM

Sorghum is a truly ancient grain. There is evidence of early humans eating sorghum as far back as the last Ice Age, which could mean that early people were eating sorghum 100,000 years ago! Sorghum is a medium-size round grain. Most sorghum eaten in the United States is white or light colored, but sorghum grows in a variety of colors, from white to purple to reddish brown. Unlike many other grains, sorghum does not have a tough exterior hull, so the entire grain can be eaten.

WHOLE GRAINS AT THE GAS PUMP

Not only can sorghum fuel your day by providing you with good energy, it can also fuel your car! Sorghum is used as a source of ethanol and other biofuels. Scientists are researching even more applications for this energy-rich ancient grain, but for now, when you are filling up your tank, you just might be getting some ethanol made from sorghum with your gasoline.

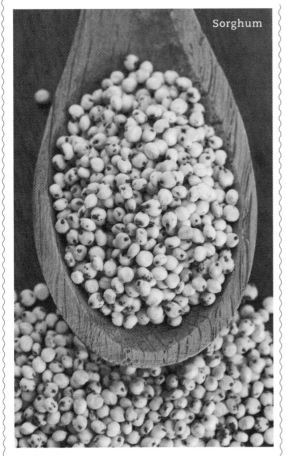
Sorghum

It is believed that sorghum originated near Egypt and then spread across Africa. Trade routes brought sorghum to India, and it probably came to the Americas via the same ships that brought slaves. Today, people all over the world rely on this nutrient-rich grain for sustenance. Like millet, sorghum is very drought resistant, making it an important crop in Ethiopia and Sudan.

The sorghum plant looks very similar to stalks of corn without the cob. Instead, sorghum has seed heads with grains the size of BB gun pellets clumped together. In the United States, not only is the grain of the sorghum plant eaten, but also the juice of the stalk is extracted to make sorghum syrup. This thick, all-natural syrup is a traditional sweetener in the southeastern United States, although it is also processed in the Midwest. The syrup is thick like molasses and can be used in place of molasses or maple syrup.

Sorghum is grown for human consumption, animal feed, and to make ethanol in the United States. In other countries, it is grown primarily for human or animal consumption.

There are many ways to enjoy sorghum. The most straightforward way is to cook the grain in water or broth and enjoy it in place of rice or pasta. It has a pleasantly chewy texture and a light flavor that works well with many different herbs and spices. Because it is gluten-free, it can be easily substituted in dishes that call for barley or bulgur.

Sorghum flour is a common addition to gluten-free flour blends or other multigrain flour blends, because it has a high protein content, a wide range of micronutrients, and a mild flavor that won't overpower baked goods. With the increased demand for gluten-free beers, sorghum has become

In the mid-nineteenth century, when West Africans were brought as slaves to America, they brought sorghum with them. The grain had long been a staple foodstuff in parts of Asia and Africa. Sorghum used for syrup, however, has a smaller seed head than sorghum that is used as a grain. Because sorghum grows so well in the South, its syrup—which is made from the juice of the stalk—became a reliable and affordable sweetener for "soul food." Today, sorghum syrup is still an important component of Southern cooking, and, because of its buttery complexity and silky finish, it is used as a substitute for corn syrup, maple syrup, honey, or molasses in recipes.

a favorite of brewers looking for a barley alternative.

Like corn, sorghum has moisture locked inside each grain. When the grain is heated in oil or a dry skillet, it will pop. The resulting popped sorghum looks like little kernels of popcorn and makes a great snack for movie night. Want to give it a try? Check out the recipe for Sorghum Popcorn (page 22).

Sorghum is slightly more expensive than millet or brown rice, so I like to make sure that I am going to use what I have. I usually buy a two-pound bag and store it in the freezer. Sorghum's chewy texture makes it an ideal vehicle for pasta sauces, when I want a change or need a gluten-free pasta alternative. I like to batch-cook sorghum and freeze it in two-cup containers so that I can pull together a quick grain salad or soup on a busy weeknight.

FARRO
(ALSO KNOWN AS EMMER)

All wheat is believed to be derived from an original ancestor, einkorn. This wild grass was originally cultivated in ancient Mesopotamia. Einkorn is a genetically simple plant with only two sets of chromosomes. Because einkorn has an inedible hull and is difficult to thresh, it was supplanted by other crops. Einkorn can be found as a specialty item, though, in well-stocked natural foods stores.

Farro is the first generation of wheat, after einkorn. It is the result of breeding (probably naturally) einkorn and goatgrass. An interesting characteristic of these types of plants is that the chromosomes get added from one variety to the other. So farro, also known as emmer, contains the chromosomes from both the original einkorn and the goatgrass with which it was cultivated.

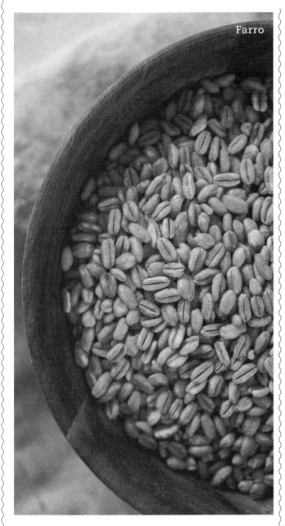

Farro

ration for soldiers in the Roman Legion.

Farro retains some of the qualities of einkorn. It is difficult to separate the inedible hull from the grain, so as hybridization continued, farro lost popularity in most of the world to its easier-to-thresh cousins. Parts of Italy have remained devoted to farro over the ages, however, and continue to enjoy this nutty grain. Elsewhere, farro is making a comeback. Some artisanal pasta makers, for example, favor flour ground from farro for pasta making, and chefs, restaurateurs, and foodies everywhere are discovering the delights of salads and other dishes that are made with this pleasantly chewy grain.

While more acreage is devoted to modern wheat than any other grain in the United States, some farmers are beginning to move to older varieties, like einkorn, farro, and

When it is ground, farro makes a finer flour than its predecessor, einkorn, which made it valuable to ancient civilizations, particularly in the Mediterranean region. It is believed that farro was a sustenance food in ancient Rome and most likely was a basic

FROM THE NEAR EAST TO ITALY AND BEYOND

Farro (or emmer) originated in the Near East and was commonly eaten in ancient Egypt. Explorers brought it to Italy, where it became an established crop. With its nutty flavor, chewy texture, and rich nutritional profile, farro is making its way onto restaurant menus and kitchen tables in the United States and around the world.

spelt. Farms in Washington, Idaho, and Montana have been growing these ancient wheats for several years, and farms in Vermont and North Dakota are exploring the option as well.

For the home cook looking for a satisfying and nutritious grain, farro is an outstanding choice. The farro that's sold in the marketplace for consumers has the hull removed; how the miller removes the hull, however, is what determines whether the farro you have purchased is a whole grain or not. Many nutrients are stripped away from pearled farro, for example, so it's important to read the ingredient label on packaging to ensure that the product is "whole farro" or "whole-grain farro."

Farro is a medium-size grain that has a warm brown color. One of my favorite ways to enjoy it is to cook it with water or broth, similar to how you cook rice, and use it as the base for grain salads. If you're short on time, you can buy quick-cooking farro that has been parboiled and is ready to eat in just 10 minutes. Otherwise, cooking a batch of farro takes less than 45 minutes. Quick Farro Risotto (page 56) is one of my favorite ways to enjoy this chewy, satisfying whole grain.

As you can do with millet and sorghum, you can also batch-cook farro and freeze the prepared grain for easy use in a recipe. I really like to use farro as a pasta alternative, so having some in the freezer, ready to go whenever I need it, can mean the difference between a healthy dinner and a convenience meal that I will regret later.

Farro's natural hull helps keep the grain from turning rancid, but the hull is partially removed from store-bought farro, so you need to keep it cold if you're not going to

AN UNWELCOME FAMILY VISITOR

Farro and spelt are the result of natural breeding in ancient times between einkorn (the earliest ancestor of modern wheat) and goatgrass in the Fertile Crescent, the region of the Middle East that curves from the Persian Gulf through modern-day southern Iraq, Syria, Lebanon, Jordan, Israel, and northern Egypt. Hybridization efforts created modern wheat. However, because wheat and goatgrass share a long history and thrive under the same growing conditions, controlling goatgrass continues to be problem for wheat growers. An invasive weed that's carried by wind and water, goatgrass spreads all too easily and is difficult to get rid of once it contaminates wheat fields, negatively impacting yield, degrading the land, and reducing farmers' profits.

use it right away. You can keep farro in the refrigerator if you're going to use it within two or three weeks or in the freezer for longer storage.

SPELT

Spelt is the result of hybridizing emmer, or farro, with another strain of goatgrass. Even if farmers may have selected plants with the best attributes to replant, spelt and farro are both considered Landrace crops, meaning they have been domesticated in the field, over time.

On the other hand, modern wheat is a product of a great deal of human manipulation, much of which was done for good reasons. Spelt and farro are tall plants, as high as four or five feet tall; modern wheat has been bred to be much shorter, around one foot tall. A shorter stalk can support a heavier seed head, so breeding short plants with more grain on each stalk produces more food. Modern wheat has also been cultivated in such a way that the hull can easily be removed from the grain during threshing, making it all the more efficient to turn grain into the flour that is used in the bread, cereal, and pasta that most Americans eat on a daily basis.

The almost universal cultivation of wheat has had a downside, however. More and more acres have been planted across the globe with this single crop—a mono crop—

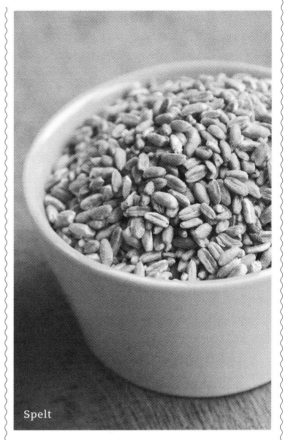

Spelt

leaving its healthy predecessors on the brink of extinction. Fortunately, the many benefits of spelt (and farro) have returned to the forefront of the natural food movement, and more and more acres are being planted with these ancient grains.

Spelt, with its taller stalks, also has a deeper root system than conventional wheat. This is important in times of drought and extreme temperatures. Deeper roots can extract nutrients and water from the soil better than shallower root systems can.

Spelt is available as a grain that can be cooked like other grains, though it needs to soak for several hours before cooking due to its tougher bran layer, unless you're using a slow cooker to prepare the spelt. In my opinion, though, spelt really shines as a whole-grain flour.

Spelt flour is available as white flour and whole-grain flour. For the former, it is processed like white wheat flour, in which the bran and the germ are removed, resulting in a white fluffy flour. This flour will work very well in place of all-purpose flour, but I think using whole-grain spelt flour is the way to go.

Whole-grain spelt flour has a lovely, light texture that makes for fantastic baked goods: whole-grain spelt cookies, cakes, and muffins have an airier texture than their counterparts made with whole wheat. When baking with yeast, whole-grain spelt flour really rises to the occasion. You can mix up a bread dough using whole-grain spelt flour, let it rise, and transfer it into the baking pan without any extra kneading or manipulation. The bread that results will have lovely air pockets and a texture that no other whole-grain bread can rival. Try Spelt Oat Bread (page 72) or Spelt Sandwich Loaf (page 73) to start baking with spelt.

Some people with gluten intolerance can better digest the proteins in spelt or farro than in traditional wheat. It is possible that the crossbreeding and hybridization that created the short, high-yield wheat plants that are so commonplace today have caused changes to gluten structures within the wheat molecules. That is one explanation why gluten intolerance seems to be so much more prevalent today than it has been in the past. If this is the case, using an ancient grain that has been less manipulated might provide a viable alternative for some people who suffer after eating modern wheat. Spelt (and farro) are members of the same family as wheat, however, so if you have a wheat allergy or celiac disease, it is still advisable to avoid spelt and farro. If you have been avoiding wheat for any medical reason, be sure to get medical advice before experimenting with any relative of wheat.

TEFF

Teff is the tiniest of the ancient grains. Each grain is approximately the size of a poppy seed. Because they are so small, you can eat the whole grain, unlike other grains that can be eaten only after the hull has been removed. Consequently, you can eat teff and enjoy all of the nutrients that are available to nourish your body.

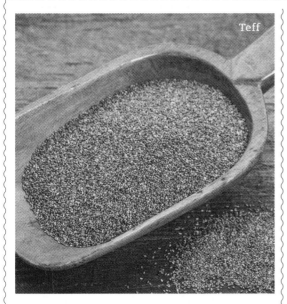
Teff

Most teff that is available in the United States is dark brown in color, but it also comes in several other shades, including ivory, golden brown, and dark reddish brown. Teff has been feeding the people of Ethiopia and Eritrea for thousands of years. Its startling ability to grow under a wide range of conditions makes it ideally suited for unpredictable climates. Teff can grow both under drought conditions and in extremely damp environments, and it can grow well at many different altitudes, as well.

A little teff goes a long way. It only takes about a handful of seeds to plant a field of teff grass. This makes it a very important crop in places with a history of food shortage. Teff's super-growing qualities have caught the attention of farmers around the world, including those in the United States and Europe, who are beginning to experiment with this versatile grain.

In Ethiopia, teff is commonly eaten as *injera*—a fermented, crêpe-like bread or pancake made from teff and water. Typically, injera is used as a surface on which other foods are piled. Diners tear off a piece of injera, wrap a bit of food inside, and then eat it with their fingers. The bread thus becomes a delicious edible utensil and serving plate all at once.

Teff should not be limited to the making of injera, however. The tiny seeds can be used to make a smooth porridge, replace cornmeal in polenta, or add crispiness to a coating for oven-fried vegetables. Teff is gluten-free and can be ground into flour for use in gluten-free flour blends. It adds a depth of flavor to vegetarian dishes, like Multigrain Veggie Burger Crumbles (page 62), and because teff is so tiny, it cooks more quickly than other ancient grains. It doesn't need to be batch-cooked, because you can make some when you need it, or you can toss it whole into a stew or soup and it will cook with the other ingredients. The protective hull is not removed, so you can store teff in your pantry, but I like to keep all of my grains in the refrigerator or freezer to maximize their freshness.

OATS

It is not clear when people started cultivating oats as food, but it is believed that oats were originally considered a weed, one that got mixed in with other grains that early people purposely harvested. There is evidence that oats have been grown as a crop to feed people and animals for over 2,000 years, if not longer.

Oats can be grown anywhere that has a cool, moist climate, which makes them well suited for cultivation in northern Europe, Canada, and the United States.

Although oats have been a breakfast staple in Scotland for hundreds of years, they were viewed as suitable food only for animals in England and elsewhere until the twentieth century. Over the past several decades, studies linking oat consumption and lower levels of blood cholesterol have brought oats front and center as a health food that offers multiple benefits.

Once people discovered the slightly sweet flavor of oats, they were hooked. Oats are processed in a variety of ways, but they are almost always sold as a whole grain, with their germ and bran intact. Even though they are cut, steamed, and toasted—to ensure a longer shelf life—all of these methods utilize the whole grain.

Oats are one of the most affordable whole grains you can buy, and rolled oats (sometimes called old-fashioned oats) are available at any grocery store. Oats are also available as steel-cut oats, which yield a chewier texture than rolled oats. Scottish oats are creamier than steel-cut, because they are cut with ceramic wheels instead of steel blades, which yields smaller pieces. Quick-cooking oats are also available, but while the result is smooth, it can also be a little gummy. The type of oats you ultimately choose depends on your taste preference and how you want to use them.

Since I cook a lot with oats, I like to buy rolled oats in at least four-pound bags. I keep them in the refrigerator, because I know that it will take me a few weeks to go through them. You can buy oats in smaller quantities or in bulk bins at most well-stocked grocery stores or natural foods stores. I use rolled oats in Nutty Granola (page 39) or to thicken smoothies and soups (see Tomato Soup, page 46). I also love cool and creamy Basic Overnight Oats (page 30) with a sprinkling of fresh berries for summer breakfasts.

I don't limit myself to rolled oats, though. In the cooler months, I make a double batch of Slow Cooker Steel-cut Maple and Brown Sugar Oats (page 34) and keep it in the refrigerator. This makes it easy to serve a portion with some warmed-up nondairy milk and a topping of dried or fresh fruit, seeds, or nuts whenever anyone wants it for

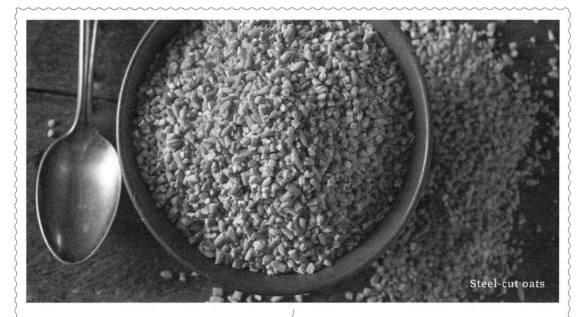
Steel-cut oats

breakfast. Each member of my family ends up with a customized breakfast that requires only a minute or two of effort. It's ideal for school days.

Versatile oats don't stop at the breakfast bowl. Oat flour is sweet, moist, and dense. I prefer to buy milled oat flour because it's finer, but I can make my own with a nut and seed grinder or a clean coffee grinder, in a pinch. If your oats are gluten-free, your oat flour will be gluten-free, too. (You can also buy professionally milled gluten-free oat flour.) Another great advantage of oat flour is that it doesn't require a binder, like xanthan gum or guar gum, to hold baked goods together, because the protein in oat flour provides structure on its own. If you don't need your flour to be gluten-free, incorporating oat flour into your baking is still a great option, because it gives a subtle sweetness to baked goods of all kinds, from muffins to cookies.

More and more people are looking for a way to limit or eliminate dairy from their diets, and oats can fill that need, too. Soaking rolled or steel-cut oats in water, then blending and straining the liquid, results in a creamy milk (page 27) that you can use as is or flavor in a variety of ways.

To learn more about these amazing ancient grains, read on! Chapter 2 explains each of their health benefits and sets the stage for cooking, eating, and enjoying ancient grains every day.

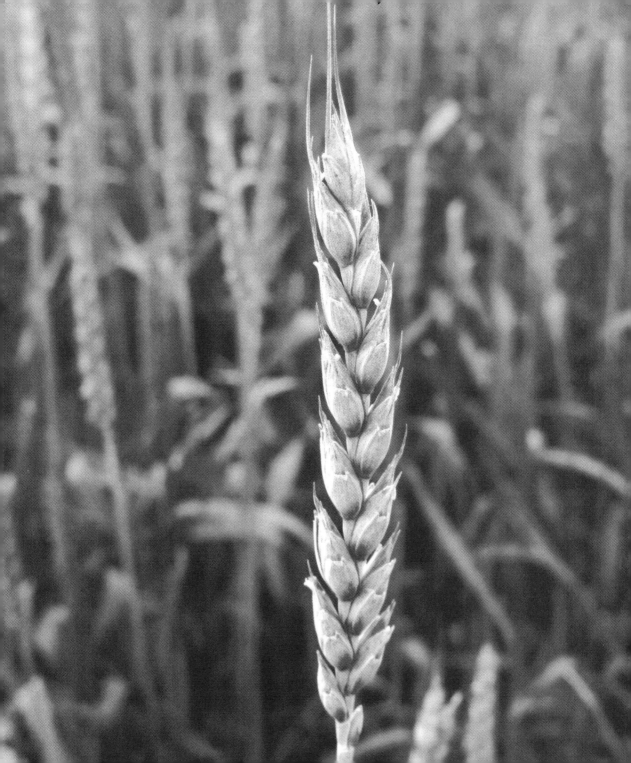

WHY WHOLE GRAINS?

Each of the ancient grains—millet, oats, sorghum, spelt, farro, and teff—contains important nutrients that your body needs to thrive. Eating them as whole grains elevates your health to even greater heights, conferring benefits that include a healthier heart and a slimmer waistline, while lowering your chances of contracting chronic diseases.

In a 2010 supplement to *The Journal of Nutrition* titled "Putting the Whole Grain Puzzle Together: Health Benefits Associated with Whole Grains—Summary of American Society for Nutrition 2010 Satellite Symposium," nutrition researchers reviewed studies looking at the benefits of whole grains from around the world. This review resulted in some clear findings about the value of eating whole grains several times a day.

Research shows that your heart benefits from eating whole grains regularly. Whole grains help to reduce cardiovascular disease in a number of ways; for instance, the fiber they contain can help eliminate excess dietary cholesterol and bile acid that can damage your arteries. Additionally, whole grains (particularly ancient grains) are rich in antioxidant and anti-inflammatory micronutrients that can have a beneficial effect on heart health. Numerous studies from Europe and North America that were part of the American Society for Nutrition symposium also found that whole grains can contribute to healthier blood pressure.

Other studies, including the landmark Framingham Heart Study conducted by Boston University and the National Lung, Heart, and Blood Institute since 1948, have shown that eating whole grains instead of refined or processed grains like white flour can decrease abdominal fat, thereby preventing a host of health problems, including a greater risk for diabetes, heart disease, and some cancers. In 2012, *The Journal of Nutrition* published a study showing that postmenopausal women who replaced refined grains with whole grains and then followed a calorie-restricted diet lost the same amount of weight as women who just followed a calorie-restricted diet but did not change to whole grains. However, the women on the whole-grain eating plan lost more abdominal fat—another strong indicator of the health advantages associated with a diet that includes whole grains.

Whole grains can play a helpful role in slimming down, and not just your abdomen. Numerous studies from around the world cited in the American Society for Nutrition summary have shown that eating whole grains in place of processed or refined grains can lower your body mass index (BMI). With the well-established health risks that come from obesity, it makes good sense, from a weight-management perspective, to incorporate whole grains into your diet on a regular basis.

Whole grains are a wonderful source of dietary fiber, as well: they contain all of the vitamins and minerals that are present in the bran, the germ, and the endosperm of the grain, whereas the process of refining grains and flours strips away the nutrient-rich bran and germ layers of the seed.

In fact, the one-two punch of fiber and nutrients in whole grains has been shown to protect against the development of chronic diseases like type 2 diabetes, cancer, and chronic heart disease. Fiber also helps your body remove waste efficiently, while the vitamins, minerals, and micronutrients present in whole grains help nourish and strengthen your body. Foods rich in fiber, like ancient grains, help you feel fuller and can help prevent you from overeating.

Think about what is marketed to American consumers—grab-and-go convenience foods, microwaveable pouches and packages loaded with chemicals and refined grains, and colorfully packaged crackers, cookies, and chips. These foods all lead to the health struggles that have become commonplace in the modern era. Obesity, heart disease, stroke, type 2 diabetes, and cancer are all on the rise. Even children are struggling with these health concerns, something that was unheard of just a couple of generations ago. Making some simple changes, like swapping out refined and processed grains for whole grains, particularly ancient grains, can set you on a healthier course. The result? You'll feel and look better than ever.

WHAT'S SO GREAT ABOUT "ANCIENT" GRAINS?

Modern grains, particularly modern wheat, have been bred and developed to provide the greatest yield with the easiest harvesting methods. Wheat strains have been selected to be dwarf varieties with larger-yielding grain heads. This hybridization process has been beneficial to a degree. More wheat, and therefore more food, is available at a lower cost than ever before. The downside to this move toward a monoculture of modern wheat, however, is that much of the wheat consumed in the United States today is refined wheat. That means that the nutrient-rich layers of the wheat are stripped away, leaving only the softer endosperm to be ground into flour. Frequently, this softer flour is enriched with vitamins and minerals before the flour is turned into the cereals, crackers, and breads on which so many people rely. The micronutrients present in the whole grain, however, are not replaced, and neither are all of the macronutrients, including fiber, along with other vitamins and minerals. Furthermore, many people report that they have trouble digesting the gluten proteins in modern wheat—proteins that have changed over time, just as the plants themselves have changed.

MILLET

Millet, a gluten-free grain, is a good source of several minerals, including copper, phosphorus, manganese, and magnesium. Manganese and phosphorus are both important for bone health and can help you better absorb calcium, another important nutrient for strong bones. The copper in millet contributes to healthy red blood cells and a healthy nervous system. Like all of the ancient grains, millet is a good source of dietary fiber and boasts six grams of protein per cup of cooked grain. Millet is also rich in antioxidants and can provide protective effects against some cancers. Eating foods rich with whole-grain millet, as opposed to refined flours, can help prevent type 2 diabetes.

SORGHUM

Sorghum is also a gluten-free grain and is as good a source as millet for many of the same nutrients, including manganese, phosphorus, and fiber. Sorghum is also a good source of selenium and niacin (also known as vitamin B3). Selenium is very important in keeping the immune system working properly, while niacin, a water-soluble vitamin, is important for healthy skin, digestion, and a healthy nervous system. Because niacin is water-soluble, your body doesn't store it, so you need to get a regular supply from the food you eat. Sorghum, like millet, is also rich in antioxidants, which can play a part in reducing the risk of some cancers.

OATS

Oats are truly a superfood. They are a good source of protein, fiber, and many minerals, including iron, magnesium, phosphorus, zinc, copper, manganese, and selenium. Oats are also a good source of thiamine (also known as vitamin B1). Thiamine plays an important role in making energy available from the carbohydrates you eat and is essential for a healthy nervous and muscular system. Oats are rich in soluble fiber, and this fiber has been shown to decrease LDL, the so-called "bad" cholesterol. Decreasing LDL is important for a healthy heart, because when cholesterol accumulates in the blood it can create dangerous plaque buildups that can clog your arteries and lead to a heart attack or stroke.

FARRO AND SPELT

Both farro and spelt are ancient forms of modern wheat. When eaten in their whole-grain form, as opposed to white spelt flour or pearled farro, which are both refined versions, these wholesome grains are packed with nutrients and flavor. Spelt and farro are rich in antioxidants, which scavenge the cell-damaging free radicals that come from exposure to pollution in the environment and chemicals in the food we eat and the water we drink. Eating foods rich in antioxidants can lead to better heart health and provide protection against developing certain forms of cancer. Farro and spelt are good sources of protein, fiber, phosphorus, and manganese. The protein in farro and spelt, like that in other ancient grains, is considered an incomplete protein because it does not contain all of the amino acids (the building blocks of protein) that we need in order to thrive. However, eating other plant foods, such as beans, soy, peanuts, quinoa, and amaranth, provides the missing amino acids. You do not need to eat these complementary proteins in the same meal with farro or spelt, because your body stores them—and if you eat a variety of fruits, vegetables, legumes, and whole grains, you can get the complete proteins that your body needs.

Spelt and farro, like all members of the wheat family, contain gluten. Although many people can safely digest gluten, others must avoid eating it and therefore cannot eat farro or spelt. At present, the only treatment for people with celiac disease, an autoimmune disease, is to avoid eating gluten completely. Even trace amounts can cause painful and/or unpleasant symptoms, and long-term exposure can cause a host of health problems. For others with a condition called gluten intolerance or non-celiac gluten intolerance, symptoms range from digestive discomfort to debilitating pain. Interestingly, some people who have gluten intolerance (not celiac disease) say they can tolerate the gluten in farro or spelt, but not the gluten in modern wheat. If you have a gluten intolerance, check with your doctor before trying these ancient versions of modern wheat. If you have celiac disease, do not eat spelt or farro.

TEFF

Teff is a grain on the rise. Long eaten in Ethiopia and Eritrea, this protein-rich tiny grain is also a good source of calcium, something that's unusual for a grain. Because teff is so tiny, it is always eaten as a whole grain—it would be very difficult to remove the bran or germ from such a little grain. Teff is also gluten-free, so its demand is increasing across the world as more people clamor for gluten-free, nutrient-rich grains. Teff is rich in micronutrients like iron, magnesium, phosphorus, zinc, copper, manganese, thiamine (vitamin B1), and pyridoxine (vitamin B6). Phosphorus and manganese help contribute to strong bones, while pyridoxine helps with brain development and function, and iron contributes to healthy blood.

The healthiest diets are richly varied. Micronutrients that are abundant in one grain might be lacking in another. Modern diets that rely so heavily on one grain—wheat—prevent that diversity. Incorporating ancient grains like millet, teff, spelt, farro, sorghum, and oats into your diet is a terrific way to ensure that you are getting a wide range of nutrients. The chapters that follow are full of great ideas for basic grain preparations as well as recipes for breakfast, lunch, dinner—and even snacks and dessert—that will help make it easy and delicious to incorporate healthy whole grains into your diet. Here's to your health!

WHICH ANCIENT GRAINS ARE GLUTEN-FREE?

Gluten is a protein that is present in some cereal grains, including wheat, rye, and barley. Because spelt and farro are related to modern wheat, they also contain gluten. Millet, sorghum, oats, and teff are all naturally gluten-free. Because of cross-contamination, which can occur anywhere along the line from the field to the packager, it is important to look for the circular "Certified Gluten-Free" label on packaging if you need to avoid gluten for health reasons, even with grains that are otherwise labeled "gluten-free."

CHAPTER 3

BASIC RECIPES FOR ANCIENT GRAINS

One of the most straightforward ways to ensure good nutrition is to eat a wide variety of whole foods—lots of different fruits, vegetables, legumes, and whole grains. It's a little shocking when you take a look at the grains—or should I say, the grain—that has taken over our kitchens. From that one look, you'd never know that there are grains other than wheat to be had: for so many of us, mornings start with a wheat flake cereal, followed by a sandwich made with whole wheat bread for lunch, then a wheat flour pasta for dinner— and don't forget all the wheat-based treats like pretzels and cookies that can be munched on throughout the day! Adding diversity to your diet is as easy as incorporating a few ancient grains into your menu. The first step—learning how to make basic preparations—is as easy as making rice on your stove top. In fact, cooking millet produces a fluffy grain that can take the place of rice in your favorite recipes; or you can serve it hot, as a silky-smooth breakfast cereal.

You'll also discover that old-fashioned oats, a breakfast staple in so many of our kitchens, can be ground into a nutrient-dense, gluten-free flour or transformed into a nourishing nondairy milk. Spelt can be cooked in a slow cooker overnight to become a toothsome side dish or the centerpiece of a main dish, or it can be milled into a wonderful whole-grain flour to make fluffy breads that don't require kneading. Tiny teff cooks up into the consistency of polenta, with an earthy flavor that you will love. Teff can also be ground into versatile gluten-free flour and used as a crunchy breading. Cooked sorghum is delightfully chewy, and uncooked sorghum can be popped as easily as corn—and it tastes just as good. Farro is another versatile grain that brings a nutty heartiness to salads and can take the place of pasta, topped with your favorite sauce.

Getting to know these ancient grains will start you on a path that will make your body and your senses happy.

PREPARED SORGHUM

MAKES 2½ CUPS

Chewy, delicious sorghum is a hardworking super grain in the kitchen. You can use it to substitute for farro, spelt, or barley whenever you need a sturdy gluten-free grain. Sorghum is rich in protein, iron, and fiber, without the gluten that can be problematic for folks with gluten sensitivities. Whether you need a gluten-free grain or not, you will be glad to know this delicious grain.

1   cup (200 g) sorghum grain

3   cups (750 mL) water or vegetable broth

1. Rinse the sorghum, place in a pot with the water or broth, and bring to a boil.

2. Cover and reduce heat. Simmer until tender, approximately 50 to 60 minutes.

3. Drain the excess liquid.

CHEWY WHOLE GRAINS

One of the best things about whole grains is their chewy nuttiness. Farro, spelt, and sorghum are all large grains that have a toothsome bite, and, because they are similar, you can substitute one for the other. Easily make a farro recipe gluten-free by substituting sorghum. You can also use sorghum in recipes that call for barley or wheat berries.

SORGHUM POPCORN

MAKES 1 CUP

Of course, there are a lot of important nutritional reasons for eating ancient grains, but they also can be fun to eat. Popping sorghum, just as you would popcorn, gives you a new way to enjoy this whole grain. You still get all the health benefits while munching on this tiny, crunchy snack. Just like popcorn, it can be eaten plain, lightly salted, or dressed up with a variety of spices. I like to enjoy sorghum popcorn with a light dusting of smoked paprika, nutritional yeast, and sea salt. My family also really likes sorghum popcorn sprinkled with gluten-free tamari.

1   tablespoon olive oil

2   tablespoons sorghum grain

1. In a medium saucepan, heat the olive oil and 2 or 3 sorghum grains over medium heat.

2. When the grains pop, add the remaining grains and cover. Shake the pan as the grains pop.

3. When the popping slows down, remove the pan from heat.

SLOW COOKER SPELT

MAKES APPROXIMATELY 5 CUPS

Spelt flour is one of my favorite whole-grain baking flours, but you are cheating yourself if you use spelt only in its milled form. Spelt grains, or spelt berries, as they are sometimes called, cook up with a nutty flavor and a toothsome texture. Pairing spelt with a favorite sauce elevates the whole dish, transforming it into a filling and satisfying entrée.

2   *cups (400 g) spelt berries*
6   *cups (1.5 L) water or vegetable broth*

1. In a slow cooker, combine the spelt berries and water or broth. Cover and cook on high for 4 hours or on low for 6 to 8 hours.

2. Drain the excess liquid.

FOR A CHANGE OF PACE

Spelt can be used in place of farro or sorghum in any of the recipes in this book. And, since spelt can take a fair amount of time to cook, my favorite way to prepare it is in my slow cooker on low overnight. All I need to do in the morning is drain the cooked spelt, pop it into the refrigerator, and heat it up in the evening with a hearty pasta sauce for a quick weeknight dinner. If you batch-cook spelt, you can freeze extra portions for future use.

SPELT, STOVE-TOP METHOD

MAKES APPROXIMATELY 2½ CUPS

If you don't have a slow cooker, you can still enjoy spelt's chewy texture and nutty flavor. Spelt cooks best if it soaks for 8 hours, or overnight. Drain the soaking liquid before you cook the spelt. If you don't have broth on hand, you can toss a bouillon cube into the cooking water for extra flavor.

3   *cups (750 mL) water or vegetable broth*
1   *cup (200 g) dry spelt berries, soaked for at least 4 hours, or overnight*

1. In a large pot, bring the water or broth to a boil.

2. Add the spelt berries, stir, and cover. Reduce the heat and simmer for 45 to 60 minutes, or until the grains are chewy.

3. Drain the excess liquid.

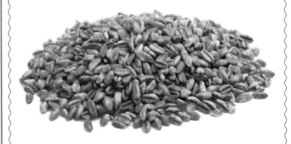

BASIC MILLET

MAKES 2½ CUPS

Cooked millet is fluffy, with a slightly chewy texture. It can take the place of rice in your favorite recipes and makes a lovely gluten-free stand-in for couscous. Millet is similar in size and color to couscous, so it can bring your favorite Mediterranean and Middle Eastern recipes back to the menu, if you've had to give up gluten. I like to cook millet in broth for savory applications, but I cook it in water when I'm making sweeter recipes, like Coconut Millet Pudding (page 93).

1 cup (200 g) millet

2 cups (500 mL) water or vegetable broth

1. In a small saucepan, combine the millet and water or broth. Bring to a boil.

2. Stir, cover, and reduce the heat to low. Simmer for approximately 20 minutes, or until the liquid is absorbed.

3. Remove from the heat and let stand, covered, for another 10 minutes. Fluff with a fork before serving or using in another recipe.

BASIC FARRO

MAKES APPROXIMATELY 2 CUPS

Farro is making its way onto restaurant menus for good reasons. For one, it anchors grain salads, allowing other flavors to shine, while providing a hearty, wholesome base. Farro can take the place of pasta in main dishes, too, giving them a rustic flare, and you can serve it as a comforting side dish. I love this ancient grain topped with a creamy sauce in Farro and Cashew Cream Sauce (page 65). And, just as is possible with other grains in this book, you can make a big batch of farro and freeze the extra to use whenever you like. You are then ready to quickly prepare a meal that has all the ease of a convenience food, along with the nourishment of ancient grains.

1 cup (200 g) farro

3 cups (750 mL) water, vegetable broth, or stock

1. In a medium saucepan, combine the farro and water or broth.

2. Bring to a boil, reduce heat to medium-low, and simmer for 30 minutes, or until the farro is tender.

3. Drain off any excess liquid.

BASIC TEFF

MAKES 1½ CUPS

Tiny teff makes for a smooth grain porridge with a nutty flavor and a mighty nutrient punch. Because teff is rich in calcium and iron, it can take the place of polenta and provide a very nutritious side dish. I love the depth of flavor that teff adds to vegetarian dishes, making them feel more substantial. Teff-Lentil Sloppy Joes (page 63) are appealing to all kinds of eaters.

  2 *cups (500 mL) water*
  ½ *cup (100 g) teff*

1. In a medium saucepan, bring the water to a boil.

2. Add the teff. Cover, reduce the heat, and simmer for 15 to 20 minutes, or until the liquid is absorbed.

TINY TEFF

Teff is one of the tiniest of edible grains. One grain of teff is about the size of a poppy seed. In fact, teff is so tiny that in one gram there are 3,000 teff grains!

OAT FLOUR

MAKES APPROXIMATELY 1 CUP

Although you can make any ancient grain into flour, the best one for gluten-free baking is oat flour. It contains similar proteins to the gluten in wheat flour, so the molecules hold together when oat flour is used in baking, just as they would with wheat flour. Other gluten-free flours require a binder like xanthan gum, guar gum, or psyllium when used in baking; otherwise the finished product is too fragile. If you need a small amount of another ancient grain flour for baking, you can follow the same procedure explained below. Please note, though, that spelt and farro are very hard grains, and it will be difficult to grind flour that is fine enough for baking, unless you have a flour mill. The finer the flour, the better the result will be for any ancient grain. If you use oat flour that you've ground yourself, the cookie and muffin recipes in this book will have a chewier texture and might be a little flatter than baked goods made with milled flour. I bake a lot with oat flour, so I buy commercially milled oat flour regularly. If I need a small amount and have run out of it, then I grind my own.

  1 *cup (80 g) rolled oats or (180 g) steel-cut oats*

1. Grind thoroughly in a blender, nut or seed grinder, or clean coffee grinder.

OTHER HEALTHY USES FOR OATMEAL

REMEDY FOR ITCHY SKIN

Oatmeal comes to the rescue when you have itchy skin. Whether your skin is dry from winter weather or you're suffering from sunburn, good old-fashioned oats can soothe your discomfort. The secret to an effective oatmeal bath is to use finely ground oats (like oat flour) in your bath water. This will make the water milky and let the oats do their soothing work. If the ground oats are too big, they will sink to the bottom of your tub, and you won't get the benefits of an oat bath. Once you have one to two cups of finely ground oats (the perfect amount for a full bath), sprinkle them into the tub, under the running tap, and stir the water with your hands periodically to make sure the oats are well mixed into the water. To get the most relief, keep the water temperature down. A too-hot bath will add to the irritation your skin is already feeling. It's up to you if you want to rinse off any residue from your skin before getting out of the tub. Gently pat yourself dry when you are finished, drain your tub through a drain screen, and wipe out your tub. This natural soak is not only soothing for your skin, but it's easy on your wallet, too, thanks to the affordable price of oats.

MAKE YOUR OWN MOISTURIZING SOAP

Would you like to have the skin-softening advantages of oats in your soap but still control the ingredients? You're in luck! It's easy to make your own bars of oatmeal soap. I start with my favorite soap that I buy at the grocery store. It has few ingredients and is made primarily from saponified coconut oil. To turn your favorite soap into an oatmeal soap, all you need to do is melt the bar in a pot over a medium flame or in the microwave, and stir a couple of tablespoons of finely ground oatmeal or oat flour into the melted soap. Then pour the mixture into a soap mold (or other silicone mold) and let it harden. Another way to make your own oatmeal soap is to buy a glycerin soap base from a craft store, melt the desired amount in a pot over medium flame or in the microwave, add any essential oils if you like (lavender is nice), and stir in some finely ground oatmeal. Then pour the soap mixture into a mold to harden. This makes a really thoughtful homemade gift, too.

WHAT IS COLLOIDAL OATMEAL?

When oats are used in a skin care product—soap or lotion, for example—the ingredient list includes "colloidal oatmeal." This means that the oats have been finely ground so that oat particles remain suspended in the medium instead of sinking to the bottom or floating to the top.

OAT MILK

MAKES 3 CUPS

The number of different nondairy milks that are available on grocery store shelves seems to grow every time I shop. Some of these exotic options have equally dramatic price tags. You can easily avoid shelling out big bucks for these products, however, by making your own rich, nondairy milk from oats, a perfectly affordable ancient grain. I am so grateful to know how to turn this pantry mainstay into oat milk—it saves me tons of aggravation if I'm planning a meal and suddenly realize that one of my boys drank the last of the milk earlier in the day! Making my own oat milk also allows me to customize the texture and flavor, depending on my needs. If I need a creamy beverage, all I have to do is cut down on the water. I like to add plain oat milk to my coffee, and my boys enjoy it as a drink with a little bit of vanilla and a touch of sweetener.

1 cup (80 g) rolled oats or (180 g) steel-cut oats

3 cups (750 mL) water

1. Soak the oats for 1 to 8 hours (or overnight) in enough water to completely cover the oats. Steel-cut oats will need a longer soaking time than rolled oats.

2. After soaking, drain the oats and combine with the water in a blender.

3. Blend thoroughly until the oats are completely broken down.

4. Strain the oat milk using a nut-milk bag or a fine-mesh strainer lined with a coffee filter. Press the pulp down with the back of a spoon to remove all the liquid.

5. Store the oat milk in a lidded glass jar in the refrigerator for up to 3 days, or you can freeze it in clean ice cube trays, then transfer the frozen cubes to a freezer-safe bag or container for later use.

6. Shake the oat milk before using.

FROZEN OAT MILK CUBES

The next time you make a batch of oat milk, make a little extra and pour it into an ice cube tray. When the oat milk is frozen, transfer the cubes to a freezer-safe container—perfect for making a cooling, nutritious smoothie whenever the spirit moves you. I like to blend frozen oat milk with some fresh or frozen fruit for a vitamin-packed snack my kids are sure to like. Some of our favorite fruits to include are mangoes, pineapples, strawberries, blueberries, and bananas.

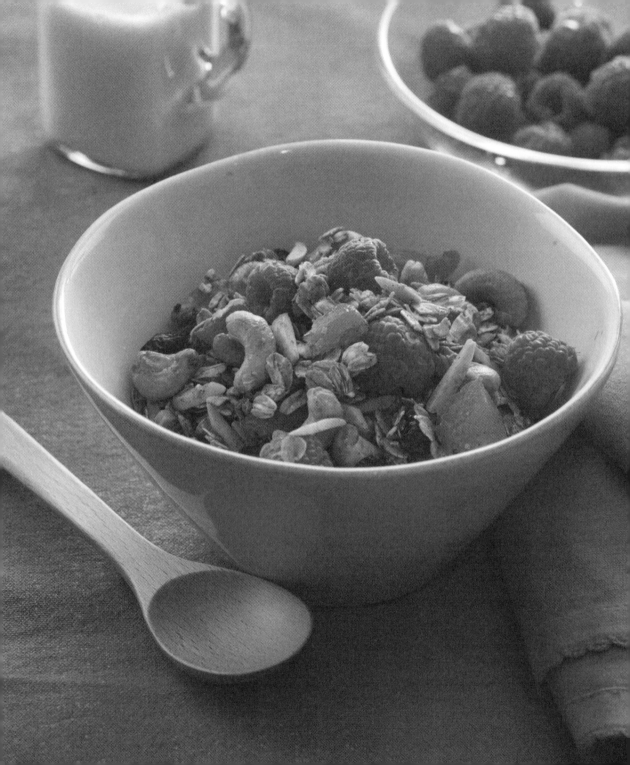

CHAPTER 4

BREAKFAST

Why start your day with cold cereal or a toaster pastry that's loaded with artificial colors and flavors when you could have something that is not only delicious, but also filled with the energy you need to begin your day? So many of the breakfast foods—muffins, cereals, and frozen waffles, for example—that have taken center stage in the past decades are made from processed, refined wheat, where all the nutrients of the whole grain have been stripped away. Some of the vitamins are put back into these products in the form of supplements, but, as we know, they do not confer the same health benefits as the real thing. Ancient grains, however, are loaded with the fiber, protein, vitamins, and minerals that naturally occur in the whole grain. They also have rich micronutrient profiles that contribute to a healthy body.

Do you prefer sweet breakfasts or are you a savory breakfast fan? For a hearty, hot breakfast, give Salsa Millet Hash (page 34), Strawberry Waffles (page 32), or Pancakes (page 31) a go. Don't have a lot of time in the morning? Prepare Peach Almond Overnight Oatmeal (page 39) for a grab-and-go breakfast when you're on the run. Nutty Granola (page 39) serves double duty as a delicious and filling breakfast cereal or as a snack to fuel you with protein, fiber, and healthy fats when you're running out of gas in the afternoon.

However you choose to enjoy your morning meal, ancient grains are easy to prepare and add diversity, flavor, and all the nutrition you need to give your day a great start.

KEYS TO GOOD HEALTH

Refined grains and flours, like white rice and all-purpose flour, have taken over Americans' kitchens—and our diet. Along with the increased availability and consumption of processed foods and refined grains, there has been a parallel surge in diseases such as type 2 diabetes and cardiovascular disease. Swapping whole ancient grains for these nutrient-void foods can indeed act as a wedge against serious health conditions and promote good health instead. Try substituting millet for white rice or whole-grain spelt flour for all-purpose flour. These subtle, easy-to-make changes in your menu can help keep you feeling your best.

OPPOSITE: **Nutty Granola, page 39**

BASIC OVERNIGHT OATS

MAKES 1 SERVING

I know why those instant oatmeal packets have survived the ups and downs of food trends over the decades—convenience. It's hard to pass up a flavorful breakfast that takes almost no time to pull together. The downside to those little pouches, though, is all the added sugar. I prefer to control the ingredients I feed my family, whenever possible. That is why I love overnight oats. I keep a stash of small lidded jars that I can set up for grab-and-go breakfasts in the morning. The kids can dress theirs up with a little maple syrup and chunky applesauce, and I can add some granola (see Nutty Granola, page 39) to mix into mine. This recipe is the basic prep for making overnight oats. The sky's the limit for how you can customize yours. Because these oats are cold, they are an ideal way to enjoy your oatmeal in warmer weather.

½ cup (40 g) rolled oats
½ cup (120 mL) nondairy milk
Fruit, nuts, seeds, or sweetener (optional)

1. In a lidded jar, combine the oats and nondairy milk.

2. Seal with the lid and refrigerate overnight.

3. Add fruit, nuts, seeds, or sweetener or enjoy plain.

MILLET PORRIDGE

MAKES 1 SERVING

On the next cool morning, change your breakfast with smooth, creamy Millet Porridge. I like to add creamy nondairy milk, such as Oat Milk (page 27), to mine. For mix-ins, dried cranberries or blueberries make an interesting alternative to raisins, and if dried fruit isn't your thing, use fresh or frozen fruit instead.

½ cup (85 g) prepared millet (page 24)
1 tablespoon maple syrup
2 tablespoons to ¼ cup (40 g) raisins
Pinch of salt
¼ teaspoon cinnamon

1. In a small saucepan, combine all the ingredients over medium heat.

2. Heat through for 3 to 4 minutes.

BATCH-COOKING TRICK

One way to pull together a healthy meal quickly is to cook a large of batch of grains. For example, make twice the amount of millet you need for a recipe and freeze the leftovers. You'll be glad you did when your family asks, "What's for dinner?" and you need only thaw the millet and add a few things to make Millet Stuffed Mushrooms (page 57) or Salsa Millet Hash (page 34).

PANCAKES

MAKES 16 PANCAKES

There is one thing I can do to be sure that my kids start their weekend happy. All I have to do is pull out my griddle pan and start making pancakes. They will eat huge piles of pancakes topped with fruit or maple syrup, or even plain. If I have any left over, I wrap them in foil and refrigerate them for a special school lunch on Monday. If you want to make your pancakes extra special, you can mix some berries, banana slices, or chocolate chips into the batter. These whole-grain pancakes have a hearty texture that holds up really well to add-ins. You can keep them warm in a 200°F oven until they are all ready to be served at one time.

1¼ cups (130 g) oat flour

1¼ cups (150 g) whole-grain spelt flour

¼ cup (35 g) evaporated cane juice or coconut palm sugar

2½ teaspoons baking powder, divided

2 teaspoons baking soda

¼ teaspoon salt

½ cup (125 g) applesauce

2¼ cups (530 mL) nondairy milk

2 tablespoons neutral oil (sunflower, grape-seed, or canola)

1 teaspoon vanilla extract

Oil for the skillet

1. In a medium bowl, whisk together the flours, sugar, 2 teaspoons baking powder, baking soda, and salt.

2. In a large bowl, combine the applesauce with the remaining ½ teaspoon baking powder. Mix in the nondairy milk, oil, and vanilla.

3. Add the flour mixture to the applesauce mixture. Stir until just combined.

4. Lightly oil a skillet or griddle. Heat until a drop of water dances on the surface.

5. Pour a generous portion (about ¼ cup) of batter into the skillet.

6. Cook until bubbles form on the surface. Flip the pancake and cook on the other side.

7. If you want to keep the pancakes warm and serve them all at once, lay the pancakes on a parchment-lined baking sheet in a 200°F oven while cooking the remaining ones.

ANCIENT GRAINS IN THE MORNING

How can you get your ancient grains when you don't have time to cook? Lots of cold cereals also feature ancient grains—millet, oats, and sorghum. You can still get all of the health benefits of these ancient grains in your bowl when you go with one of these convenient breakfast options.

STRAWBERRY WAFFLES

MAKES 10 WAFFLES

When I make waffles, I like to serve them straight from the waffle iron to the plate while my family waits (not so patiently) at the table. Everyone wants the first waffles, but someone will have to wait. If you want to serve all the waffles at the same time, preheat your oven to 200°F and lay them flat on a baking sheet until they are all done.

3   *tablespoons flaxseed meal or ground flaxseed*

¼   *cup (60 mL) warm water*

1   *cup (100 g) oat flour*

1   *cup (120 g) whole-grain spelt flour*

1   *teaspoon salt*

2   *teaspoons baking powder*

¼   *cup (50 mL) coconut oil, gently melted*

2¼ *cups (530 mL) nondairy milk*

1   *tablespoon vanilla extract*

1   *cup (150 g) sliced strawberries*

1. Preheat the waffle iron.

2. In a small bowl, combine the flaxseed meal and water. Set aside.

3. In a large bowl, whisk together the flours, salt, and baking powder.

4. Mix in the flaxseed meal slurry, coconut oil, nondairy milk, and vanilla.

5. Mix the strawberries into the batter. Stir until thoroughly combined.

6. Follow the waffle maker instructions to cook the waffles until golden brown on the outside.

DON'T DELAY ENJOYING YOUR STRAWBERRIES

Strawberries are not only a sweet summer treat, they are exceptionally good for you, too. They are high in vitamin C, manganese, fiber, antioxidants, and a variety of minerals. In order to maximize the nutritional benefits of these juicy treats, though, it's important to enjoy your berries right away. Strawberries start to lose nutritional value two days after they're picked.

PORTABLE OATMEAL

MAKES 15 PATTIES

One of the reasons why there is such a booming business in energy bars and processed breakfast pastries is because they are convenient. Everyone has had mornings where time slips by way too quickly, and you have to get out the door, leaving little, if any, time to make a meal. Instead of skipping breakfast, which will make you crabby and low on energy, you need something that you can grab and go. As lovely as a bowl of oatmeal is, it can make a mess on your shirt as you're running out the door. I came up with this recipe as a way to get the benefits of oatmeal without creating an accident waiting to happen. Portable Oatmeal is baked, so the outside is dry and firm while the inside stays soft and oatmeal-ish. You can eat this healthful breakfast on your walk to the train or in your car without spilling porridge everywhere. Did I mention how delicious it is, too?

3   *cups (700 g) of prepared oatmeal that has been refrigerated for at least 1 hour or up to 2 days*

1   *cup (250 g) chunky applesauce*

¼   *cup (40 g) shelled hemp seeds (hemp hearts)*

Sprinkling of cinnamon

1. Preheat the oven to 375°F (190°C/gas mark 5). Line two baking sheets with parchment paper.

2. In a large bowl, combine the prepared oatmeal with the applesauce and hemp seeds.

3. Scoop ¼ cup of the oatmeal mixture and shape it into a round patty. Place on a baking sheet.

4. Repeat with the remaining mixture.

5. Sprinkle the patty tops with cinnamon.

6. Bake for 45 to 50 minutes, or until the outside of each patty is firm and golden.

7. Refrigerate for up to four days or freeze the patties for up to three months.

8. Warm the patties in the toaster, oven, or microwave before enjoying again.

WHICH IS BETTER FOR YOU— STEEL-CUT OR ROLLED OATS?

No matter which style of oats you choose—rolled oats or steel-cut oats—you'll enjoy health benefits from almost the same nutritional profile: ¼ cup of uncooked rolled (or steel-cut) oats (20 g) boasts a full range of nutrients, including 5 grams of protein, 4 grams of fiber, and barely any sugar (rolled oats have 0 grams, while steel-cut have 0.5 grams). If you're looking for a healthy grain, whichever way you cut your oats, you've made a good choice.

SLOW COOKER STEEL-CUT MAPLE AND BROWN SUGAR OATS

MAKES 8 SERVINGS

Although cooking rolled oats takes only a few minutes, steel-cut oats can take up to 45 minutes. I am busy in the morning trying to get everybody ready for the day and don't have that kind of time. Instead, I make a big batch of steel-cut oats in my slow cooker overnight. That way, everyone in the family can wake up to the captivating aroma of maple and brown sugar and enjoy steel-cut oats right away. I refrigerate leftovers and reheat them the next day with nondairy milk (see Oat Milk, page 27). In this way, my family can enjoy a sweet breakfast treat more than once during the week, and I don't have to spend a lot of time waiting for the oats to cook!

- *2 cups (350 g) steel-cut oats*
- *8 cups (2 L) water*
- *Pinch of salt*
- *1½ teaspoons cinnamon*
- *½ teaspoon nutmeg*
- *¼ cup (25 g) brown sugar (or coconut palm sugar)*
- *¼ cup (80 mL) maple syrup*

1. In a slow cooker, combine the ingredients.

2. Cook on low for 8 hours.

SALSA MILLET HASH

MAKES 4 SERVINGS

Sometimes I prefer a savory brunch entrée instead of sweet. Salsa Millet Hash is ideal for those mornings when a sweet breakfast won't do. Millet gives this hash a fluffy texture, and the whole grain combines with fiber-rich veggies to keep you feeling full, but not weighed down, through the afternoon. Serve this savory hash with Blueberry Scones (page 75) and some fresh fruit the next time you have guests at the breakfast table.

- *1 tablespoon olive oil*
- *1 cup (150 g) finely diced Yukon Gold potato*
- *¼ cup (50 g) finely diced onion*
- *1 cup (200 g) cooked or 2 cups (100 g) raw chopped spinach*
- *2 cups (350 g) prepared millet (page 24)*
- *½ cup (100 g) prepared salsa*
- *Salt and pepper to taste*

1. In a large skillet, heat the olive oil over medium-high heat.

2. Add the potato and onion and sauté until softened, approximately 2 to 3 minutes.

3. Add the spinach and cook until wilted, approximately one minute.

4. Add the millet and salsa.

5. Cook until the millet is warmed through.

WHERE'S THE GREEN? SMOOTHIE

MAKES 2 SERVINGS

I don't keep the ingredients in my smoothies a secret from my kids. They know that I often put in spinach or kale. The blueberries in this smoothie turn this drink into a beautiful purple color, though, so they don't have to think about the spinach with every sip. The smoothie will have a smoother consistency if you presoak the oats, as called for in the directions. Don't worry if you forget, though; you can still blend them in, even if they're dry. The oats will add just a little more texture to your smoothie, but it will still taste delicious.

½ cup (40 g) rolled oats (gluten-free, if necessary)

3 cups (100 g) packed baby spinach leaves

2 cups (500 mL) apple juice

1 cup (150 g) frozen mango

1 cup (150 g) frozen blueberries

1 6-ounce (170 g) container of vanilla-flavored coconut yogurt (or other nondairy yogurt)

2 tablespoons chia seeds

1. In a large bowl, soak the oats in enough water to cover for 30 minutes or up to overnight. Drain.

2. In a blender, blend the spinach with the apple juice until the leaves are completely broken down.

3. Add the oats and blend well.

4. Add the mango, blueberries, yogurt, and chia seeds and blend until smooth.

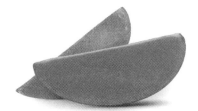

GROW A GARDEN FOR YOUR CAT

Some cats really love to eat houseplants, which can be annoying for you as well as dangerous for them. One way to keep your kitty away from your favorite plants is to grow a container garden just for her. Many cats enjoy munching on grass, particularly oat grass. Luckily—for both you and your feline friend—growing an oat grass garden is easy: just choose a container, fill it with potting soil, plant some seeds approximately ¼ inch apart, and cover them with ½ inch of soil. Water the soil and keep the container close to a sunny window. While you enjoy watching your grass grow, your cat will enjoy keeping it trimmed!

CREAMY SUNRISE SMOOTHIE

MAKES 4 SERVINGS

During the school year, smoothies are a go-to breakfast for my family. I make them at least twice a week, and frequently more often. If I know that my kids have started the day with fruits, vegetables, protein, and whole-grain oats, I don't have to stress out too much when they breeze through lunch to play outside at recess. That's why smoothies are "peace of mind in a glass" for me! Please note, if you have a high-power blender, you can cut your carrots into chunkier slices, but if you are using a standard blender, you might want to grate or shred them first to ensure they are well blended in the smoothie.

1 cup (80 g) rolled oats

3 cups (750 mL) water

1 cup (150 g) frozen strawberries

1 cup (250 g) frozen pineapple chunks

1 banana

½ cup (60 g) peeled carrot slices

½ cup (80 g) cashews or hemp seeds

1 cup (250 g) applesauce

1. Soak the oats in the water for at least 30 minutes or up to overnight. Drain.

2. In a blender, blend the oats with the strawberries, pineapple chunks, banana, carrot slices, cashews, and applesauce until smooth. For a thinner smoothie, add a little water.

KID-FRIENDLY GRAINS

As the mother of two boys, I understand how challenging it can be to give children both the nutrition they need to grow strong and healthy and also make meals and snacks that they'll actually eat! Luckily, ancient grains make it easier to create wholesome dishes that my whole family loves. Whether we're starting the day with a Creamy Sunrise Smoothie (this page) or enjoying Tomato Soup (page 46) with Spelt Flatbread (page 76) on the side for lunch, my children get the nutrients they need because they like the food. Farro and Cashew Cream Sauce (page 65) is one of our favorite comfort foods—great for dinner and packed with whole grain goodness, too. The protein in ancient grains helps your children's bodies grow strong, and the fiber will help keep their digestive systems working well. Essential minerals in ancient grains, like selenium, strengthen their immune systems, so your children have a better chance to fight off the illnesses that seem to swirl around them, in their early years, particularly at school. Ancient grains are also a good source of phosphorus and manganese—important nutrients that help build strong bones.

A WELL-STOCKED KITCHEN
FOR COOKING ANCIENT GRAINS

Preparing ancient grains doesn't require a lot of specialized kitchen equipment, but there are a few tools that will make it easier to make the most out of these superfoods. Here are some of my favorites:

- **BLENDER.** You don't need a high-power blender to create delicious smoothies and smooth soups; a good-quality standard blender will work just fine.

- **FOOD PROCESSOR.** I use a food processor to chop large quantities of vegetables, but it's also a great machine for blending doughs, such as Coconut-oil Spelt Piecrust (page 100) or Spelt Tortillas (page 76).

- **IMMERSION BLENDER.** You can use a blender for creamy soups like Tomato Soup (page 46) or Creamy Potato Millet Soup (page 45), but it's faster and easier to clean up afterward if you use an immersion blender.

- **WAFFLE IRON.** I put off getting a waffle iron for a long time. Now that I own this inexpensive appliance, I can't imagine not having it. Waffles are not only a favorite breakfast at my house, they're also a fun, quick dinner.

- **NONSTICK GRIDDLE PAN.** My griddle pan sits over two of my stove burners, and I love that I can cook several pancakes at once. I also use it to make many tortillas at a time.

- **NUT AND SEED GRINDER OR DEDICATED COFFEE GRINDER.** I like the convenience of making my own whole-grain flours, especially when I need a very small quantity. A large food processor won't grind the grains small enough, and getting out my blender can be a hassle. A small, powerful grinder does the trick beautifully.

- **GLASS JARS WITH LIDS.** I can store oat milk or any leftover smoothie or soup to enjoy later in the day.

- **FREEZER-SAFE CONTAINERS.** Batch-cooking is a sanity saver for me. I store plain cooked grains, extra portions of sauce, and soups to make meal prep easy on busy days.

EGG-FREE FRENCH TOAST

MAKES 6 SERVINGS

Substituting homemade cashew cream for eggs and milk, the traditional base for French toast, eliminates the cholesterol from this breakfast favorite, but not the flavor or texture you love. Don't limit this treat to the morning; it's a delicious option for "breakfast for dinner," too. Serve it with a Creamy Sunrise Smoothie (page 36), and your family will never suspect that you're still providing them with a nutritious meal. They'll think they tricked you into giving them a treat for dinner! And is anything better than the fragrance of vanilla and cinnamon in your kitchen? *Note:* For a gluten-free version of this recipe, you can use Multigrain Gluten-free Biscuits (page 79) in place of the bread.

1 cup (150 g) cashews or hemp seeds (for nut-free)

2 cups (500 mL) water

2 teaspoons vanilla extract

⅛ teaspoon salt

1½ teaspoons cinnamon

1 loaf of Spelt Oat Bread (page 72) or Spelt Sandwich Loaf (page 73), sliced

1. If you are using a standard blender, soak the cashews in water for 4 hours, then drain and rinse them. If you are using a high-power blender or hemp seeds, presoaking is not necessary.

2. In a blender, combine the cashews or hemp seeds with the 2 cups of water, the vanilla, salt, and cinnamon. Blend until smooth.

3. Pour the liquid into a shallow bowl.

4. Dip a slice of bread in the bowl, turning to allow both sides to soak up the liquid.

5. Lightly oil a skillet or griddle. Heat on medium-high heat until until a drop of water dances on the surface.

6. Cook the soaked bread until golden brown on both sides. Repeat with the remaining slices of bread.

CELEBRATING OATS

January is National Oatmeal Month. That's no surprise, as more oats are eaten in January than at any other time. After all, what could be better than filling, comforting, whole-grain oats to help you keep your New Year's resolution to slim down ... healthfully? This January, make a batch of Nutty Granola and celebrate one of my favorite grains. You can feel good doing it!

NUTTY GRANOLA

MAKES 3 CUPS GRANOLA, OR MORE WITH OPTIONAL DRIED FRUIT

When you bake oats with natural sweeteners, fragrant spices, and flavorful nuts, you'll want to keep the resulting granola on hand all the time. This recipe makes a super-tasty cereal and snack that has all the healthy fats, protein, complex carbohydrates, and fiber that will give you lasting energy as you go about your day. My family enjoys it served with nondairy milk or yogurt for breakfast, or as a snack later in the day. I change the dried fruits in the recipe from time to time to keep it interesting, but we almost always have a jar of granola on our kitchen counter. You can store it in a sealed glass container for up to a week.

- 2 cups (160 g) rolled oats (gluten-free, if necessary)
- ½ cup (50 g) slivered almonds
- ½ cup (80 g) cashew pieces
- ⅛ teaspoon salt
- 1 teaspoon pumpkin pie spice (or a heaping ¼ teaspoon each of cinnamon, dried ginger, and nutmeg)
- ¼ cup (60 mL) apple juice
- ¼ cup (60 mL) agave nectar
- Dried fruit of your choice—raisins, dates, apricots, blueberries, cherries, and cranberries are all delicious (optional)

1. Preheat oven to 350°F (180°C/gas mark 4). Line a baking sheet with parchment paper.

2. In a large bowl, combine all the ingredients. Spread the mixture on the baking sheet.

3. Bake for 15 minutes, or until the granola is golden brown and fragrant. Cool completely.

PEACH ALMOND OVERNIGHT OATMEAL

MAKES 1 SERVING

Once you've mastered Basic Overnight Oats (page 30), you're ready to move on to something a little fancier. Fresh peaches bursting with juice make this oatmeal a cross between a treat and a quick breakfast. Peaches and almonds are related botanically, so their flavors marry well in this dish.

- ½ cup (40 g) rolled oats (gluten-free, if necessary)
- ½ cup (120 mL) nondairy milk
- 1 to 2 drops almond extract
- 2 tablespoons slivered almonds
- 1 medium ripe peach, diced, or ¾ cup (100 g) frozen peaches, thawed and diced
- 1 to 2 teaspoons evaporated cane juice or coconut palm sugar (optional)

1. Combine all the ingredients in a lidded jar. Refrigerate overnight. Stir before eating.

COCOA POWER BITES

MAKES APPROXIMATELY 18 BITES

I like to run. It's a challenge before a longer run to know what to eat that won't weigh me down but will provide me energy to finish strong. Cocoa Power Bites are the answer! I keep a batch refrigerated and eat one or two before a run. They are naturally sweetened with dates, so I won't get the sugar crash that can result from refined sweeteners. The nut butter and coconut oil give me healthy, slow-burning fats that keep me energized over the long haul, and the fiber-rich oats keep me from feeling hungry. Try these before your next run or take some with you on a hike.

1 cup (200 g; 10 to 14) Medjool dates

½ cup (120 mL) water

¼ cup (20 g) cocoa powder

1 tablespoon coconut oil

¼ cup (60 mL) nondairy milk

½ teaspoon vanilla extract

¼ cup (60 g) sunflower seed butter or other nut butter

1½ cups (120 g) rolled oats

1. Line a baking sheet with parchment or wax paper.

2. Remove the pits from the dates. Press the dates firmly into a 1-cup measuring cup until you have a full cup.

3. In a food processor, puree the dates and water into a smooth paste.

4. In a medium saucepan over medium heat, combine the date paste, cocoa, coconut oil, and nondairy milk, stirring continuously for 3 minutes.

5. Remove the mixture from the heat and mix in the vanilla, sunflower seed butter, and oats.

6. Drop the batter by the tablespoonful onto the lined baking sheet. Chill in the refrigerator at least 1 hour.

7. Transfer the bites to a sealed container stored in the refrigerator. The bites should keep for 1 week.

POWER UP YOUR WORKOUTS WITH ANCIENT GRAINS

Munching a couple of Cocoa Power Bites before a workout or hike is a great way to fuel up, but plenty of other ancient grain recipes in this book provide you with quality energy to get the most out of your exercise routine. For example, you can spread almond butter or sunflower seed butter on a slice of toasted Spelt Oat Bread (page 72) and top it with a few slices of banana, or if you grab a couple of Portable Oatmeal patties (page 33), you have a treat that won't weigh you down. And a Creamy Sunrise Smoothie (page 36) is another delicious choice.

CINNAMON MUG COFFEE CAKE

MAKES 1 SERVING

I am crazy about single-serving cakes, a preference that luckily keeps me from eating the lion's share of a cake that's big enough for the whole family. Instead, with this recipe, I can quickly pull together ingredients for a mini cake, pop it into the microwave, and enjoy just enough of a delicious treat without any leftovers for later indulgence. I usually have all the ingredients for this little coffee cake on hand, so if I'm stuck for an idea for breakfast, I can make it quickly. If you don't have oat flour for this cake already in your pantry, you can easily grind your own (see page 25 for instructions). It will work well here. Make sure that you really combine the dry and wet ingredients when you're preparing this cake—you don't want the last bites to taste powdery.

5   tablespoons oat flour (gluten-free, if necessary)

Pinch of salt

¼   teaspoon cinnamon

¼   teaspoon baking powder

2   tablespoons applesauce

2   tablespoons maple syrup

1   tablespoon water

1. In a microwave-safe coffee cup or small bowl, whisk together the flour, salt, cinnamon, and baking powder.

2. Mix in the applesauce, maple syrup, and water until completely combined. (Make sure that all the dry ingredients are incorporated.)

3. Cook in a microwave on high for 1 minute; or, if you're using an oven, bake the mixture in a 350°F (175°C/gas mark 4) preheated oven for 10 to 15 minutes, or until a toothpick inserted into the center of the cake comes out clean.

WINDY CITY COCOA

As the mom of a child with food allergies, I know firsthand the need to say, "No, you can't have that." I have worked for years to broaden the world for people living with restricted diets by providing recipes that are safe for many different dietary needs. I have long relied on ancient grains to help create safe and alternative treats. One of my favorite ancient grains—oats—stars in my newest creation, Windy City Cocoa. Windy City Cocoa is a dairy-free instant hot cocoa. It gets its creaminess from whole-grain gluten-free oats, bringing the joy of hot cocoa to people with dairy allergies, and to vegans and folks who are gluten-free. An added bonus of using oats in the mixture is that not only is it a hot cocoa, it's also a cake mix.

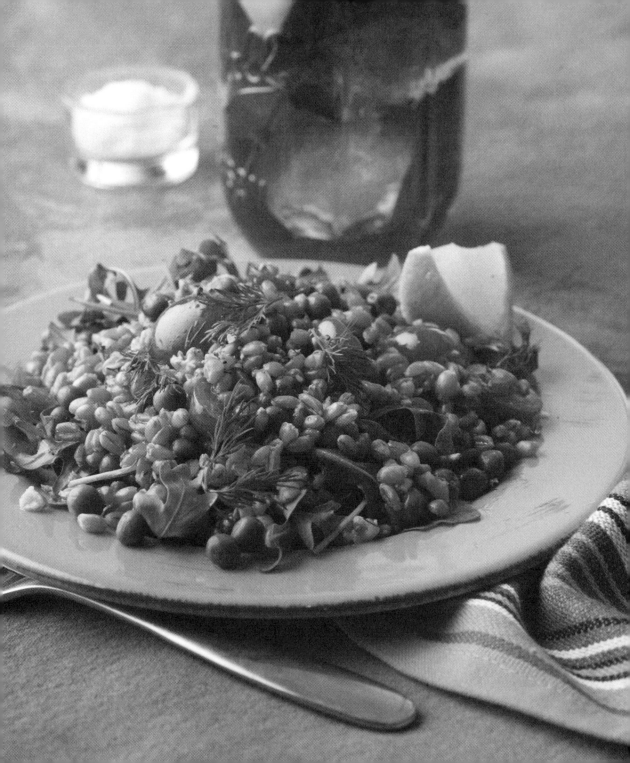

CHAPTER 5

SOUPS AND SALADS

Ancient grains have a place at every meal, including in soups and salads. If you can't have mushroom barley soup because you're gluten-free, that's not a problem, because Mushroom Sorghum Soup (page 44) is so fragrant and earthy, you'll be slurping up mushroomy goodness by the bowlful. In fact, the earthy flavor of ancient grains pairs beautifully with a wide range of vegetables, taking them to new heights. For example, if you never thought you could enjoy a creamy soup without the addition of dairy, look no farther than the recipe for Tomato Soup (page 46), where oats supply all the silky creaminess you want without the added cholesterol, or hearty Creamy Potato Millet Soup (page 45) that delights with the lingering, comforting texture of millet. In fact, all the soups in this chapter are good for satisfying your soul, just as a piping hot bowl of soup should—and they make an ideal lunch to fuel a productive afternoon, thanks to fiber-rich ancient grains.

In the summertime, when farmers' markets are bursting with produce, ancient grains help round out hearty veggie salads, keeping hunger at bay and energizing your day. Whether you'd like a main dish salad for a warm summer evening or a cool, simple side salad to complete the meal, ancient grains bring flavor, texture, and nutrients to your favorite cold dishes. Lemon Dill Grain Salad (page 48), for example, is a lovely recipe that can be customized any way you like, with sorghum, farro, or spelt. To add a nice crunch to a fruit-laced greens-based salad, try using croutons made from ancient grain flatbreads (page 76). You'll never use the store-bought stuff again!

KEEP YOUR ANCIENT GRAINS COOL

Although you can store your grains in a covered container in the pantry, I prefer to keep my grains in the freezer or refrigerator to extend their shelf life. The fats in the grains can cause them to go rancid when exposed to heat or if kept at room temperature for too long. Because I like to vary the grains that I'm cooking with on a weekly or monthly basis, I can easily have half a bag of a grain that I might not use again for a couple of weeks. If I store it in the freezer, I know that it will still be fresh even if I don't use it for two or three months.

OPPOSITE: **Lemon Dill Grain Salad, page 48**

MUSHROOM SORGHUM SOUP

MAKES 6 SERVINGS

Mushrooms make me think of fall; there is something soul-satisfying about them. This soup builds on dried mushrooms that are ground into a powder and used to flavor the broth, along with button mushrooms, which are sliced and added to the soup. Sorghum adds chewy texture and, because it's a gluten-free grain, everyone can enjoy it. For a delicious accompaniment, try Garlic Flatbread (page 78) or Multigrain Gluten-free Biscuits (page 79).

1   ounce (30 g) dried mushrooms
    (I like porcini)

2   tablespoons olive oil

1   leek, white and light green portions,
    thoroughly washed and thinly sliced,
    about ¼ cup (20 g)

1   teaspoon dried thyme

1   cup (250 mL) white wine

8   cups (2 L) water

1   cup (200 g) rinsed sorghum grain

3   cups (200 g) thinly sliced
    button mushrooms

Salt and pepper to taste

1. In a food processor or blender, grind the dried mushrooms. Set aside.

2. In a large soup pot, heat the olive oil over medium heat.

3. Add the leeks, thyme, and dried mushrooms and sauté for 2 minutes, until the vegetables have softened.

4. Add the white wine and bring to a boil; allow to boil for 2 minutes.

5. Add the water, sorghum, button mushrooms, and salt and pepper to taste.

6. Return to a boil, cover, and reduce the heat. Simmer for 45 minutes to 1 hour, or until the sorghum has softened.

SORGHUM SYRUP

Sorghum syrup is the result of juice that has been extracted from sorghum and then boiled down. It is a natural sweetener that can be used in place of maple syrup, corn syrup, or molasses. To replace one of these sweeteners with sorghum syrup in cooking or baking, substitute one for one with sorghum syrup. Due to the availability and marketing of these other sweeteners, sorghum syrup was out of fashion after the 1970s. With renewed interest in ancient grains, however, this liquid sweetener is becoming more popular again.

CREAMY POTATO MILLET SOUP

MAKES 8 SERVINGS

This is a thick, creamy soup, but it doesn't use any dairy or even nondairy milk. Instead, it gets its creaminess from starchy millet and potatoes. If you prefer a slightly thinner soup, use water or extra stock to thin it down a bit; if you have leftovers, simply add a little extra liquid when reheating.

1   *tablespoon olive oil*

1   *medium onion, small dice (approximately 1 cup)*

2   *cloves garlic, minced*

1   *cup (200 g) millet*

10 *cups (2.5 L) vegetable stock, plus more if needed*

1   *teaspoon salt (unless stock is already salted)*

1   *teaspoon Dijon mustard*

10 *Yukon Gold potatoes with skin, cut into 2-inch chunks (about 5 cups)*

Sliced scallions for garnish

1. In a large stockpot, heat the olive oil over medium heat.

2. Add the onion and garlic and sauté for 2 to 3 minutes, or until they begin to soften.

3. Add the remaining ingredients, except scallions.

4. Bring to a boil, reduce the heat, and simmer for 35 to 45 minutes, or until the potatoes are very tender.

5. Blend the soup with an immersion blender in the pot, or transfer the soup in batches to a blender and blend until smooth.

6. Thin with water or additional stock to the desired consistency, as this soup is thick. Serve immediately and garnish with scallions.

TOMATO SOUP

MAKES 6 SERVINGS

Creamy tomato soup is the definition of comfort food, especially this one, which gets its creaminess from an unexpected source—oats! You won't taste the oats, though, just the bright flavor of tomatoes with the perfect amount of seasoning. If you want a spicier soup, add a dash of Tabasco or Sriracha to fire it up. Alongside, serve a couple thick slices of Spelt Sandwich Loaf (page 73). Perfection!

- 1 cup (80 g) rolled oats
- 1 cup (250 mL) water
- 1 tablespoon olive oil
- 1 medium red onion, diced (approximately ½ cup)
- 3 cloves garlic, minced
- ½ teaspoon dried thyme
- 2 28-ounce (about 800 g each) cans San Marzano or plum tomatoes with basil
- Salt and pepper to taste

1. Soak the oats in the water for at least 4 hours, or until the water is absorbed by the oats.

2. In a large saucepan or stockpot, heat the olive oil over medium-high heat.

3. Add the onion and garlic and sauté for 2 to 3 minutes, or until softened but not browned. Add the thyme and stir to combine.

4. Add oats, tomatoes, and salt and pepper to taste. Reduce the heat to medium-low and cook for 20 minutes, stirring occasionally.

5. Blend the soup in the pot with an immersion blender, or transfer the soup in batches to a blender and blend until smooth.

MILLET AND POBLANO CHILI

MAKES 6 SERVINGS

This chili packs quite a kick, which I love, but if you prefer a milder dish, you can substitute some or all of the poblano peppers with green bell peppers. If you make this chili in the morning, it will be perfect heated up later for a game-day meal. Serve it with some Spelt Tortillas or Flatbreads (page 76), which you can toast and crumble into croutons to add some crunch. I like to serve this excellent chili with chopped avocado, too.

- 2 tablespoons olive oil
- 1 medium onion, diced (approximately ½ cup)
- 3 cloves garlic, minced

3 small to medium poblano peppers, seeds and ribs removed, and minced (approximately 2 cups, or 200 g)

1 teaspoon dried thyme

1 teaspoon dried oregano

⅓ cup chili powder

2 bay leaves

½ teaspoon salt

1 cup (175 g) prepared millet (page 24)

1 28-ounce (about 800 g) can crushed tomatoes

1 15-ounce (about 400 g) can kidney beans, drained and rinsed

1. In a large pot, heat the olive oil over medium-high heat.

2. Add the onion, garlic, and peppers and sauté, stirring, for 3 minutes, or until soft and fragrant but not browned.

3. Add the thyme, oregano, chili powder, bay leaves, and salt and stir until incorporated.

4. Add the millet, tomatoes, and beans and stir well.

5. Reduce the heat and simmer for 45 minutes, stirring occasionally.

6. Remove the bay leaves before serving.

MIX-AND-MATCH SALADS

Mason jar salads—salads that are layered in a glass jar with a lid that you shake before eating —are all over the Internet, and for good reason. Who doesn't love a lunch that you can put together the night before you need it? Salads in a jar are wonderfully versatile because they can be made from an infinite number of ingredients, each with its own flavor and texture. You'll never get bored, because you can change what goes into your lunch every day. Ancient grains are right at home in Mason jar salads, whether you're using cooked sorghum, millet, oats, teff, spelt, or farro, and they'll help you feel satisfied and energized all afternoon. How do you make one of these salads? Start by layering the wettest ingredients in the bottom of the jar so that any fragile ingredients (like leafy greens) won't get soggy. I like to use a vinaigrette or salsa on the bottom, but any dressing is a good option. On top of that, add cooked grains and then a layer of heartier vegetables or fruit, like beets, raisins, or radishes. Now you're ready for the last and most delicate layer—lettuce, micro greens, fresh herbs, etc. Cover the jar with a tight lid, and when you're ready to enjoy your salad, give the jar a gentle shake. This will coat all of the ingredients with just the right amount of dressing. Don't forget to add nuts, seeds, fruit (especially berries), and veggies to your salad jars—variety will help keep you interested in eating the healthy stuff!

LEMON DILL GRAIN SALAD

MAKES 4 SERVINGS

A substantial grain salad like this one makes a nice change from the usual pasta or potato salad. Any chewy ancient grain will work well, whether farro, spelt, or sorghum. If you choose sorghum, your salad will be naturally gluten-free. This fresh-tasting salad is also a terrific option to pack for a picnic, because it's filling and tastes best when served at room temperature.

4 cups (800 g) prepared sorghum, spelt, or farro (pages 22–24)

1 cup (150 g) fresh peas

1 cup (150 g) grape tomatoes, halved

¼ cup (60 mL) plus 2 tablespoons fresh lemon juice

2 tablespoons olive oil

2 tablespoons minced fresh dill

Salt and pepper to taste

1. In a large bowl, combine the farro, peas, and tomatoes.

2. In a small, lidded jar, shake together the lemon juice, olive oil, dill, and salt and pepper to taste.

3. Pour the dressing over the salad and toss.

GREEN SALAD WITH FLATBREAD CROUTONS

MAKES 2 SERVINGS

In my opinion, green salads are best when they incorporate a wide range of flavors and textures. This salad delights with crunchy croutons, toothsome sunflower seeds, crisp greens and carrots, and tender, sweet kiwis. Serve this salad, using your favorite (or mixed) greens, alongside spicy Millet and Poblano Chili (page 46) to provide a cooling contrast.

FOR THE SALAD

2 Spelt Tortillas or Flatbreads (page 76)

4 cups (80 g) mixed salad greens

¼ cup (35 g) sunflower seeds

½ cup (65 g) diced cucumber

¼ cup (25 g) shredded carrots

1 kiwi, peeled and sliced

FOR THE VINAIGRETTE

¾ cup (180 mL) olive oil

¼ cup (60 mL) balsamic vinegar

¼ teaspoon salt

¼ teaspoon pepper

2 teaspoons agave nectar

1. To make the salad, toast the tortillas or flatbreads until crispy and crumble them into 1-inch pieces.

2. In a large bowl, toss the croutons with the salad greens, sunflower seeds, cucumber, carrots, and kiwi.

3. To make the vinaigrette, place the oil, vinegar, salt, pepper, and agave nectar into a lidded jar. Shake well.

4. Pour the vinaigrette over the salad, toss, and serve.

BRUSSELS SPROUTS MILLET SLAW

MAKES 2 SERVINGS AS A MAIN DISH OR 4 SERVINGS AS A SIDE DISH

Shredded Brussels sprouts make a sturdy base for this satisfying salad. You can find shredded or shaved Brussels sprouts in the produce section of well-stocked supermarkets, but you can also make your own in a food processor or with a mandoline—they'll look as pretty as they taste. Brussels sprouts are an excellent source of vitamin K, which you need for healthy blood.

FOR THE SLAW
1   cup (50 g) shredded Brussels sprouts
½   cup (50 g) shredded carrots
½   cup (85 g) prepared millet (page 24)
¼   cup (30 g) dried cranberries
¼   cup (35 g) sunflower seeds

FOR THE DRESSING
1   tablespoon agave nectar
1   tablespoon Dijon mustard
2   tablespoons apple cider vinegar
1   tablespoon olive oil
Salt to taste (optional)

1. To make the slaw, combine all the slaw ingredients in a large bowl.

2. To make the dressing, whisk together all the dressing ingredients in a cup or small bowl.

3. Pour the dressing over the slaw and toss.

ENJOY YOUR PRODUCE STRAIGHT FROM THE FARM

Whether you're enjoying a crisp summer salad, a rich and comforting winter soup, or a vibrant fruit dessert, the best dishes rely on high-quality ingredients. One of the ways to bring that extra-special something to your cooking is to use farm-fresh produce. When fruits and vegetables come directly from the farm to your table, you can practically taste the sunshine. To get all the health and flavor benefits of those straight-from-the-farm fruits and vegetables, shop at your local farmers' market or join a CSA (Community Supported Agriculture). To find a farmers' market or CSA near you, visit LocalHarvest.org and type in your zip code. You'll be surprised to find what's growing nearby!

ROASTED VEGETABLE SALAD WITH APRICOT-DIJON VINAIGRETTE

MAKES 2 SERVINGS AS A MAIN DISH OR 4 SERVINGS AS A SIDE DISH

Don't be scared off by the cooked radishes in this salad. Roasting brings out a sweetness in radishes that balances their natural bite. This is a salad that you will love to make all fall and winter long, when cruciferous vegetables like cauliflower and broccoli are available. Sorghum gives a chewy textural contrast to the crunchy vegetables, and the apricot-kissed dressing brings just the right amount of sweetness to this beautiful salad. Serve it with a Multigrain Gluten-free Biscuit (page 79) or a Savory Drop Biscuit (page 81).

½ medium head cauliflower

1 medium bunch broccoli

8 radishes

2 tablespoons olive oil

½ teaspoon salt, plus more to taste

¼ cup (35 g) pepitas (shelled pumpkin seeds)

1 tablespoon apricot preserves (I use an all-fruit variety)

1 tablespoon apple cider vinegar

1 teaspoon Dijon mustard

1 cup (180 g) prepared sorghum (page 22)

1. Preheat the oven to 400°F (200°C/gas mark 6).

2. Chop the broccoli and cauliflower florets into 1-inch (2.5 cm) chunks. Cut the radishes into quarters.

3. Toss the vegetables with the olive oil and ½ teaspoon salt.

4. Bake on a parchment-lined baking sheet for approximately 15 minutes, checking after 10 minutes for doneness. The vegetables are done when they are easily pierced with a knife but are not very brown.

5. Toast the pepitas in a dry skillet over medium heat for approximately 2 minutes, shaking them frequently. The pepitas are done when they're fragrant and have a light golden tinge.

6. In a small bowl, whisk together the preserves, vinegar, Dijon mustard, and salt to taste.

7. Pour the dressing over the roasted vegetables and sorghum, toss, and top with the toasted pepitas.

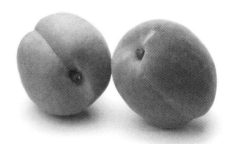

MILLET TABBOULEH

MAKES 8 SERVINGS

Tabbouleh is a delightful Middle Eastern salad that features mint and parsley combined with fresh vegetables. Traditionally, it is made with bulgur, a form of wheat. Here, millet steps in to make this fresh, vibrant salad gluten-free. Serve a scoop of Millet Tabbouleh alongside Hummus Arugula Flatbread (page 68).

1 cup (175 g) prepared millet (page 24)

½ cup (7 g) mint leaves, chopped

1 bunch flat-leaf parsley, chopped

1 medium tomato, diced
   (approximately 1 cup, or 200 g)

1 large cucumber, peeled and diced
   (approximately 1 cup, or 150 g)

3 scallions, white and light green portion,
   sliced (approximately ¼ cup, or 25 g)

⅓ cup (70 mL) olive oil

¼ cup (60 mL) lemon juice

Salt to taste (optional)

1. In a large bowl, mix the millet, mint, parsley, tomato, cucumber, and scallions.

2. In a small bowl, whisk together the olive oil and lemon juice. Season to taste with salt, if desired. Pour the dressing over the salad and toss.

3. Let the salad rest for 1 hour before serving to allow the flavors to meld.

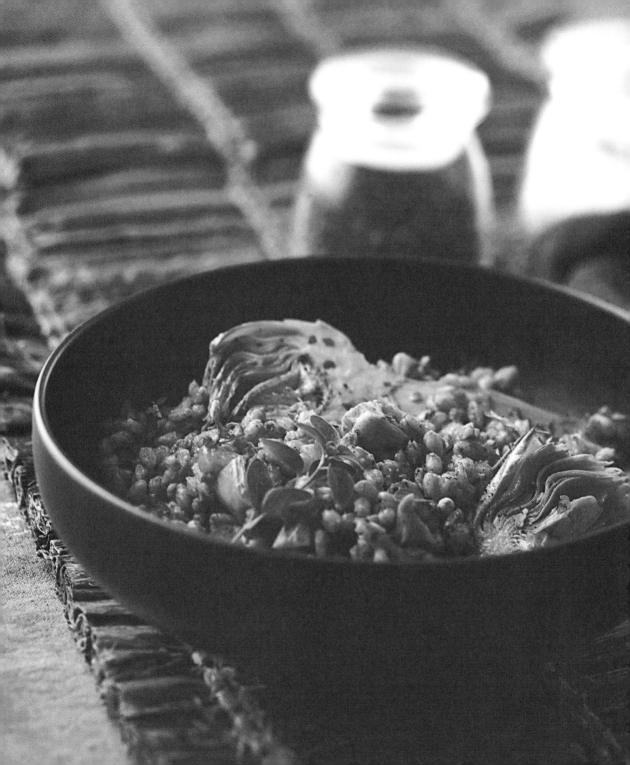

CHAPTER 6

ENTRÉES FOR LUNCH AND DINNER

Filling, versatile, and flavorful, ancient grains are ideal for the most sophisticated entrées as well as more workaday meals that need to be prepared quickly without compromising flavor or nutrition. As you'll discover in this chapter, there are so many reasons to use ancient grains in your cooking. For one, grains like teff, sorghum, farro, millet, and even the familiar oat complement flavors from all over the world—a real plus as regional flavors cross borders and arrive in our kitchens, literally giving us a taste of other places and cultures. For example, Spanish Millet (page 59) and Quick Farro Risotto (page 56) offer a taste of the Mediterranean, while Sorghum Tacos (page 55) bring some Latin American spice to the dinner table. American favorites get a healthy remake with ancient grains, too. Teff-Lentil Sloppy Joes (page 63) and Chickpea Hemp Veggie Burgers (page 69) might sound exotic, but they taste like childhood favorites.

On those evenings when you have very little time to get something on the table, ancient grain entrées come to the rescue. You can make A Quick and Easy Whole-Grain Pasta (page 67) with a Simplest Pasta Sauce (page 61) in well under an hour. Batch-cooking ancient grains also saves a tremendous amount of time, allowing you to quickly pull together Potato Millet Croquettes (page 58) or Farro or Sorghum with Bell Pepper Cashew Sauce (page 60) for a quick supper the whole family will enjoy.

When you cook an ancient grain entrée for company, rest assured that you are not only providing your guests with something interesting and delicious to eat, you are also giving them all the benefits of the protein, fiber, vitamins, and minerals that are abundant in the dish. Your guests won't even think about the health benefits when they ask for a second helping of delightful entrées like Stuffed Mushrooms (page 57) or Asparagus Sorghum Sauté (page 54). Another bonus is that almost all of these recipes can be made gluten-free, if necessary.

OPPOSITE: **Artichoke Farro, page 66**

ASPARAGUS SORGHUM SAUTÉ

MAKES 2 SERVINGS

Asparagus is one of my favorite vegetables when it's in season. I try to eat it in as many ways as possible while it's at its peak. Sautéing asparagus with mushrooms and serving it with filling sorghum (or farro, if you prefer) makes for a warming dinner on those nights when spring still has a nip in the air. You can enjoy this dish all year long by substituting the asparagus with almost any green vegetable that is in season. It works equally well with zucchini, fresh or frozen peas, and green beans. When reheating leftovers, add some extra water or broth.

1 tablespoon olive oil

2 cups (150 g) sliced button mushrooms

1½ cups (200 g) asparagus, tough ends removed and discarded, and the remaining stalks sliced into 1½-inch (4 cm) pieces

1 cup (180 g) prepared sorghum (page 22)

¼ cup (150 g) Savory Nutty Topping (recipe follows)

Freshly ground pepper (optional)

1. In a large skillet, heat the olive oil over medium heat.

2. Add the mushrooms and asparagus and sauté for 3 to 4 minutes, or until the mushrooms soften and start to release their juices.

3. Stir the sorghum into the vegetables. Cook until the asparagus is tender, approximately 3 to 5 minutes.

4. Serve in bowls and top with Savory Nutty Topping and freshly ground pepper.

SAVORY NUTTY TOPPING

MAKES OVER 1 CUP

This topping is a delicious addition to pasta dishes, steamed vegetables, or other grain dishes.

½ cup (50 g) raw sliced almonds*

½ cup (50 g) raw cashews*

¼ cup (15 g) nutritional yeast

½ teaspoon salt

¼ teaspoon garlic powder

*Or you can use 1 cup (100 g) of either almonds or cashews instead of a mix.

1. In a food processor, blend all ingredients until well ground.

2. Store in a lidded jar for 3 to 4 weeks in the refrigerator.

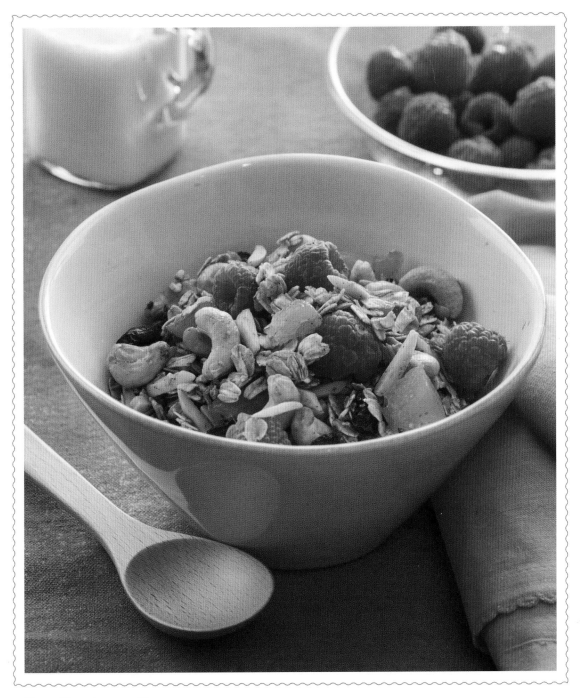

Nutty Granola, page 39

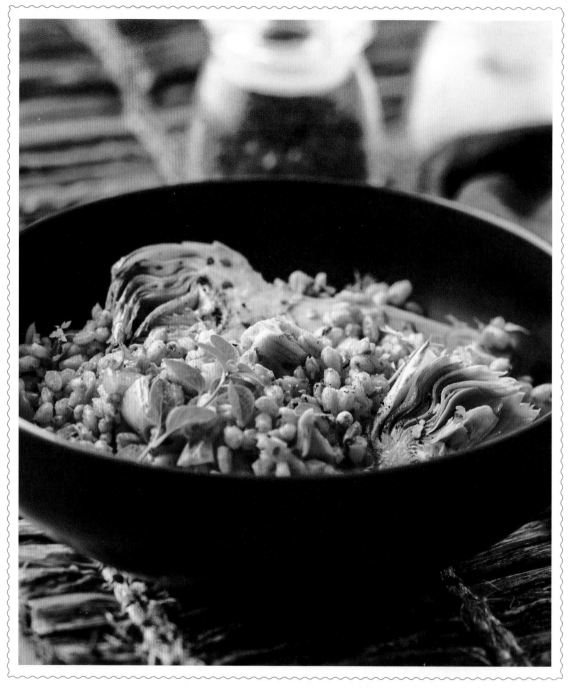

Artichoke Farro, page 66

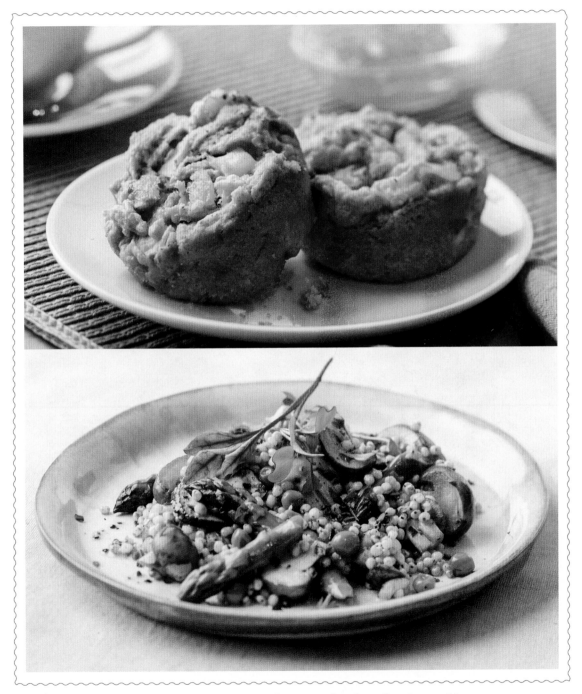

TOP: Peach Mango Muffins, page 82   BOTTOM: Asparagus Sorghum Sauté, page 54

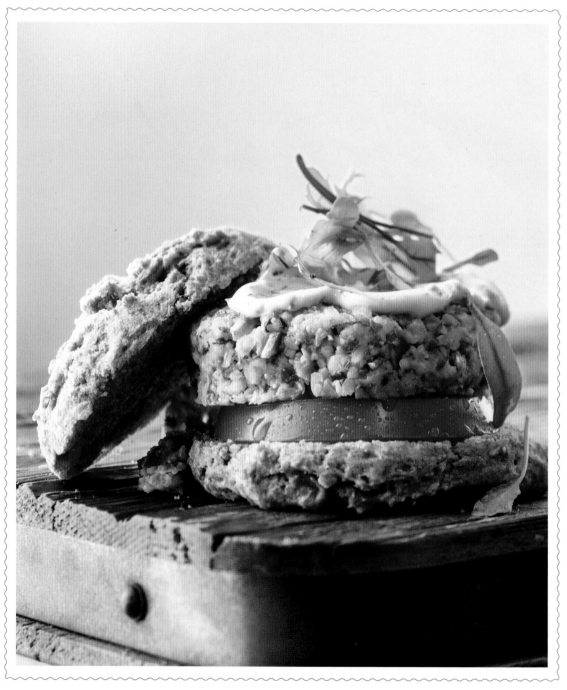

Chickpea Hemp Veggie Burgers, page 69, with Savory Drop Biscuits, page 81

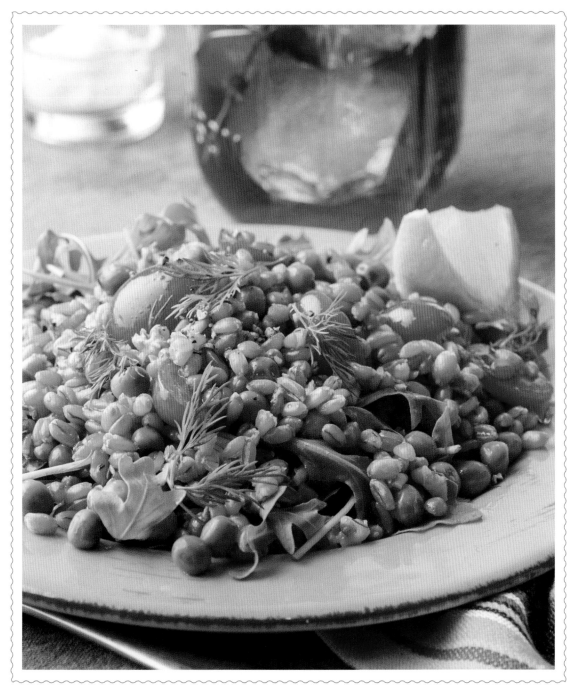

Lemon Dill Grain Salad, page 48

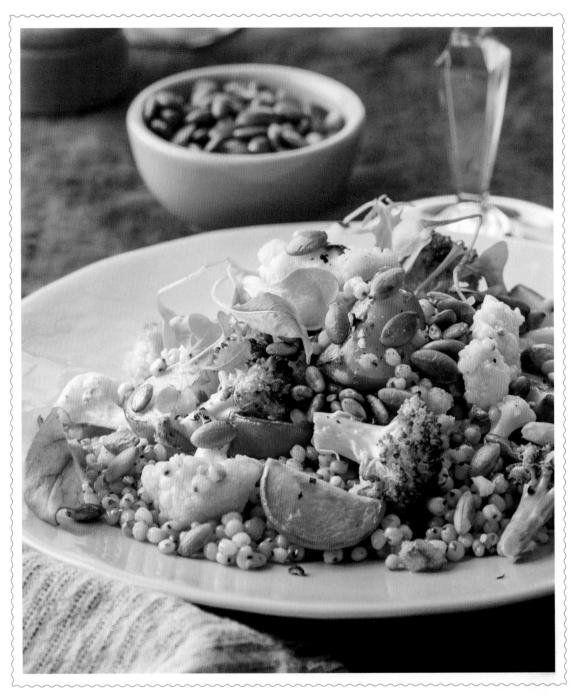

Roasted Vegetable Salad with Apricot-Dijon Vinaigrette, page 50

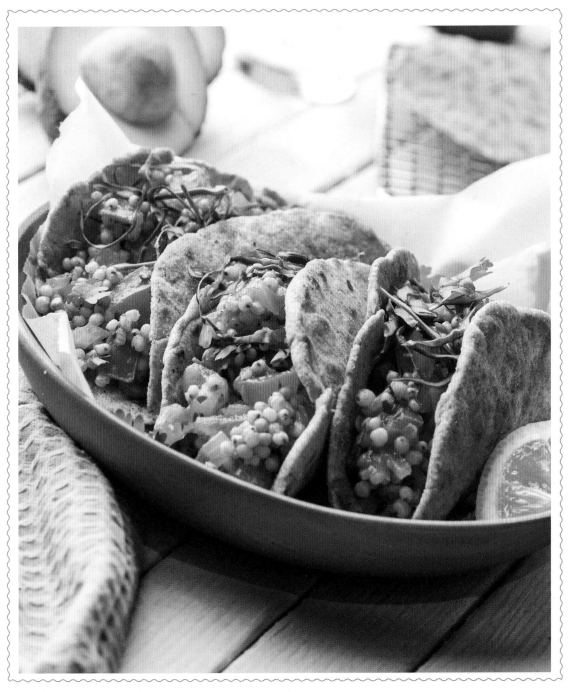

Sorghum Tacos, page 55, with Spelt Tortillas, page 76

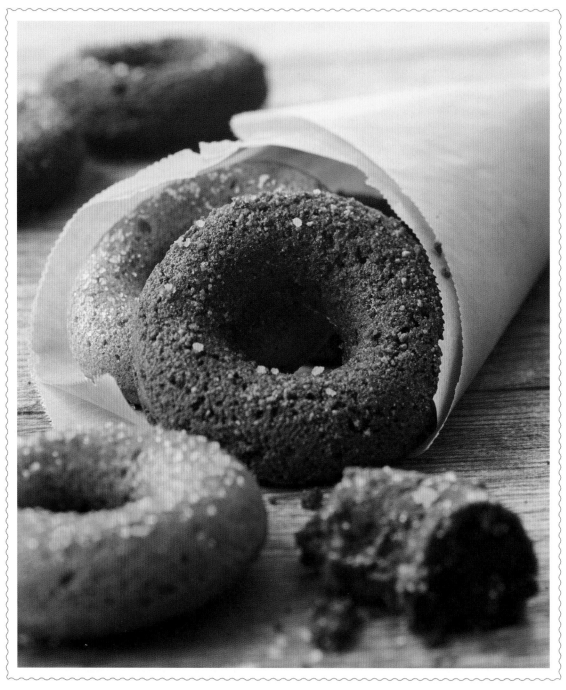

Chocolate Donuts, page 96, and Pumpkin Donuts, page 97

SORGHUM TACOS

MAKES 4 SERVINGS

In this recipe, sorghum takes an unexpected direction, replacing traditional proteins to create a flavorful taco that has a delightful texture. You can substitute millet in place of sorghum, if you prefer, and still have a delicious dish. I like to put out a mini buffet of fresh toppings to accompany these tacos—chopped cilantro, shredded red cabbage, and sliced avocado are some favorite options. You can double up on ancient grains if you serve Spanish Millet (page 59) with the tacos.

1   *tablespoon olive oil*

¾   *cup (120 g) diced onion*

2   *cloves garlic, minced*

1   *chipotle pepper in adobo sauce, minced*

2   *teaspoons tomato paste*

1   *teaspoon oregano*

1   *tomato, cored and diced*

1   *tablespoon apple cider vinegar*

2   *cups (360 g) prepared sorghum (page 22)*

8   *tortillas or taco shells*

1. In a large skillet, heat the olive oil over medium-high heat.

2. Add the onion and garlic and sauté for 2 to 3 minutes, until softened but not browned.

3. Add the pepper, tomato paste, oregano, tomato, and vinegar. Cook for 3 to 4 minutes.

4. Add the sorghum and stir to combine. Cook until heated through.

5. Serve in tortillas or taco shells.

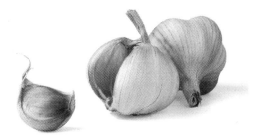

NUTRITIONAL YEAST VS. BAKING YEAST

Nutritional yeast is an ingredient that is frequently found in vegetarian and vegan recipes. It provides a nutty, cheesy flavor without using actual dairy products. Nutritional yeast is a single-celled organism (*Saccharomyces cerevisiae*) that is sometimes grown on molasses and then deactivated through drying. It is safe to eat on its own, although it is usually consumed with other ingredients or as a supplement. Baking yeast, a substance that gives rise to baked goods, is a live organism and is not safe to eat on its own.

QUICK FARRO RISOTTO

MAKES 4 SERVINGS

Traditional risottos are made with Arborio rice (a white rice) and stirred slowly as they absorb the cooking liquid. This version replaces the white rice with farro, a whole grain, and uses prepared farro to speed up the process. The personality of the finished dish is similar to a risotto—it's a wine- and herb-infused comforting dish. Knowing that you can make a risotto quickly will keep this dish in your regular rotation, rather than saving it for special occasions. If you need to eat gluten-free, you can substitute sorghum for the farro in this dish. If you have leftovers, add a little water or broth when reheating. Enjoy a glass of the leftover wine with this risotto.

- 2 tablespoons olive oil
- 8 ounces cremini mushrooms (approximately 2 cups, 140 g, sliced)
- 2 cloves garlic, minced
- ½ teaspoon dried thyme
- ½ teaspoon dried rosemary
- 1 bay leaf
- 4 cups (800 g) prepared farro (page 24)
- 1 cup (150 g) peas (fresh or frozen)
- ¼ cup (60 mL) good-quality white wine
- ¼ teaspoon salt

1. In a large sauté pan or stockpot, heat the olive oil over medium heat.

2. Add the mushrooms and sauté for 3 to 4 minutes, until they start to release their juices.

3. Add the garlic and sauté for 1 minute, or until fragrant but not browned.

4. Add the thyme, rosemary, salt, and bay leaf and sauté with the mushrooms and garlic to release their flavors.

5. Add the farro, then add the peas and wine.

6. Cook, stirring occasionally, until the liquid is mostly absorbed. The farro should still be moist, but not soupy.

7. Remove the bay leaf before serving.

MIGHTY MUSHROOMS

Incorporating mushrooms into your diet makes good sense. They are low in calories and fat, but high in fiber. Mushrooms are a good source of vitamins and minerals, including thiamine, riboflavin, niacin, pantothenic acid (vitamin B5), phosphorus, potassium, copper, and selenium. For optimal nutrition, store mushrooms in the refrigerator and use within six to eight days after buying. Do not keep mushrooms on the counter or in a pantry. Use the mushrooms before they begin to darken and get hard.

STUFFED MUSHROOMS

MAKES 12 TO 15 MUSHROOMS

I don't think I can adequately express my love for these millet-stuffed mushrooms. When I first made them, I ate way too many. Then I had to make them again right away for our annual Oscar party. They were a hit! You can serve these stuffed mushrooms as an appetizer or as a main dish and even turn them into a special-occasion meal by using portobello mushroom caps instead of smaller mushrooms. If you serve a salad, like Green Salad with Flatbread Croutons (page 48), and Savory Drop Biscuits (page 81) or Multigrain Gluten-free Biscuits (page 79) with these delicious mushrooms, you'll have a meal that's fit for a celebration.

12 to 15 mushrooms

1 tablespoon plus 1 teaspoon olive oil, divided

¼ cup (40 g) diced onion

2 cloves garlic, minced

¼ teaspoon dried dill

¼ teaspoon dried thyme

⅛ teaspoon dried sage

¼ teaspoon salt

2 tablespoons white wine

¼ cup (10 g) chopped spinach

½ cup (85 g) prepared millet (page 24)

1. Preheat the oven to 350°F (180°C/gas mark 4).

2. Clean the mushrooms and remove the stems. Mince the stems.

3. In a large skillet, heat 1 teaspoon olive oil over medium heat.

4. Add the onions, mushroom stems, and garlic. Sauté for 2 to 3 minutes, until softened but not browned,.

5. Add the dill, thyme, sage, salt, wine, spinach, and millet. Thoroughly combine and remove the skillet from the heat.

6. Place the mushroom caps top side down in a pie plate or cake pan. Place a portion of the filling inside each mushroom cap, dividing evenly.

7. Brush the remaining 1 tablespoon olive oil on top of the filling, dividing evenly.

8. Bake for 45 minutes to 1 hour, or until the mushrooms are cooked through.

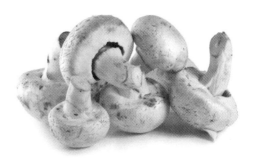

POTATO MILLET CROQUETTES

MAKES 7 CROQUETTES

Potatoes and millet make a great, natural pair. Millet's fluffy texture blends in particularly well with potatoes—in fact, you can easily mash them into potatoes (delicious!). And the combination of manganese-rich millet and potassium-rich potatoes results in a dish that's full of nutrients, including B vitamins, protein, and fiber. These croquettes make a lovely light meal when paired with a green salad, or a heartier repast when served with a bowl of Tomato Soup (page 46). You can make a double or even triple batch of these croquettes and freeze them for later meals. They will stay fresh in your freezer for at least three months. To enjoy them later, all you need to do is thaw and heat them in a 375°F (190°C/gas mark 5) oven until they're heated through.

6   *Yukon Gold potatoes*

½   *medium yellow onion, small dice (approximately ½ cup, or 80 g)*

1   *cup (175 g) prepared millet (page 24)*

½   *teaspoon dried dill or ½ tablespoon fresh dill*

½   *teaspoon salt*

Freshly ground pepper to taste

2   *tablespoons olive oil*

1. Cut the potatoes into quarters. Put them into a large saucepan and add enough water to cover.

2. Bring to a boil, then reduce to a simmer. Cook until the potatoes are easily pierced with a fork.

3. Drain the potatoes and mash with a potato masher or large fork.

4. In a large bowl, mix the mashed potatoes with the millet, dill, salt, and pepper to taste.

5. Form the mixture into ¼-cup (approximately 7 equal-size) patties.

6. Cook on a lightly oiled skillet or griddle pan over medium-high heat until browned on both sides, about 3 to 4 minutes per side.

SINGING MILLET'S PRAISE

Millet is an important crop to the indigenous people of Taiwan, where varieties of millet have long been a staple and also hold a place of honor in rituals. The Bunun people, for example, are famous for their sophisticated eight-part choral music. Recordings of the Pasibutbut, a chant for the harvesting of millet, show off this beautiful and moving style of singing.

SPANISH MILLET

MAKES 5 SERVINGS

This is a recipe for basic Spanish Millet (as opposed to Spanish Rice), which I use as a base and then add ingredients to suit my mood. Some favorite add-ins are sautéed poblano peppers, sautéed green bell peppers, corn, chopped tomato, and black beans. You can make a delicious meal with Spanish Millet as the base—just layer Spanish Millet into a bowl with sautéed greens, black beans, and chopped avocado, then top it with some chopped tortilla chips and salsa.

- 1   teaspoon neutral oil (sunflower, grape-seed, or canola)
- ¼   yellow onion, small dice
- 2   cloves garlic, minced
- 1   6-ounce (170 g) can tomato paste
- 2   cups (350 g) prepared millet (page 24)
- Salt and pepper to taste
- Water or vegetable broth, as necessary (up to ¼ cup, or 60 mL)

1. In a large saucepan, heat the oil over medium-high heat.

2. Add the onion and garlic and sauté until soft but not browned, approximately 2 to 3 minutes.

3. Add the tomato paste, millet, and salt and pepper to taste and stir to combine.

4. If needed, add water or broth, 1 tablespoon at a time, to achieve the desired texture.

HERBED MILLET

MAKES 4 SERVINGS

Herbed millet is a versatile side dish that can easily be elevated to an entrée with the addition of your favorite herbs, veggies, or beans—and it tastes extra delicious with a sprinkle of toasted almonds or sunflower seeds on top. I like to serve Herbed Millet instead of steamed rice with roasted seasonal vegetables for a light meal. This makes for a great change of pace and diversifies your diet at the same time.

- 2   cups (500 mL) vegetable broth
- 1   cup (200 g) millet
- 1   bay leaf
- ½   teaspoon salt
- ½   teaspoon dried oregano
- 1   teaspoon dried basil

1. Combine all the ingredients in a medium saucepan.

2. Bring to a boil. Cover, reduce the heat, and simmer for 20 minutes.

3. Remove the bay leaf and fluff with a fork before serving.

FARRO OR SORGHUM WITH BELL PEPPER CASHEW SAUCE

MAKES 6 SERVINGS

This dish was a favorite with my recipe testers. It tastes delicious and makes an interesting entrée for guests. You can make it with farro or sorghum (if you need a gluten-free option). It's an ideal dish for company when you don't have much prep time, because it comes together quickly if the grain is pre-cooked. Serve this as a one-dish meal or with a simply prepared vegetable, like steamed broccoli or sautéed spinach.

3 cups (450 g) diced red bell peppers

1 cup (250 mL) red wine

2 cloves garlic, minced

1 bay leaf

¼ teaspoon dried basil

¼ teaspoon dried oregano

¼ teaspoon salt

Freshly ground black pepper to taste

¼ to ½ teaspoon red pepper flakes (optional)

1 cup (150 g) cashew pieces, finely chopped

3 cups (600 g) prepared sorghum, spelt, or farro (pages 22–24)

1. In a large sauté pan, add the bell peppers, wine, garlic, bay leaf, basil, oregano, salt, black pepper to taste, and red pepper flakes, if using. Bring to a simmer, stirring occasionally, and cook for 20 minutes, until the bell peppers are tender but not mushy.

2. Remove the bay leaf, add the cashews, and stir to combine.

3. Top the farro, spelt, or sorghum with the pepper cashew sauce and serve.

ANCIENT GRAIN IS A PREHISTORIC GRAIN

The history of sorghum in Africa is truly ancient. In 2009, a leading archaeologist at the University of Calgary, Julio Mercader, found evidence that early Homo sapiens enjoyed grains long before anyone had previously believed. He found evidence of sorghum, and tools used to process it, in a cave in Mozambique, which led him to conclude that early humans were eating grains 100,000 years ago. He published his findings in the December 18, 2009, issue of the academic journal, *Science*.

Thanks to its high protein content—a whopping 22 grams per cup—sorghum has been fueling people in Africa for thousands of years. Its place of prominence is assured there, due its drought resistance. Sorghum can thrive in challenging environments where other plants cannot grow, making it an important crop not only in Africa, but in Asia, North America, and Central America.

SIMPLEST PASTA SAUCE

MAKES 3½ CUPS

Making your own pasta sauce can be almost as easy as opening a jar of sauce from the grocery store. This sauce is ideal combined with Multigrain Veggie Burger Crumbles (page 62) or served with Teff-breaded Eggplant Slices (page 64).

1   tablespoon olive oil

1   large clove garlic (or 2 small cloves), minced

1   teaspoon dried basil

1   teaspoon dried oregano

½   teaspoon dried thyme

1   28-ounce (about 800 g) can crushed tomatoes

Salt and pepper to taste

1. In a medium saucepan, heat the oil over medium heat.

2. Add the garlic and sauté for 30 seconds.

3. Add the basil, oregano, and thyme and stir. Cook for another 30 seconds.

4. Add the tomatoes, stir to combine, and simmer for 10 minutes (or longer if you have time for a fuller-flavored sauce).

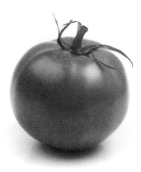

MULTIGRAIN VEGGIE BURGER CRUMBLES

MAKES 2½ TO 3 CUPS OF CRUMBLES

Teff adds depth of flavor to these veggie burger crumbles. Unlike many of the gluten-free veggie burger crumbles that you can buy at the store, these contain only wholesome ingredients. You can make a double batch and freeze half, so that you always have some ready. Veggie burger crumbles can add heft to pasta sauce; or, when mixed with salsa, they make it easy to pull together a quick meal of tacos. You can also use them to make a delicious sandwich (see Spelt Sandwich Loaf, page 73) with tomato, onion, and lettuce.

½ cup (125 g) prepared teff (page 25)

1 tablespoon olive oil plus extra for oiling the pan

¼ cup (40 g) diced onion

¼ cup (30 g) diced carrot

1 15-ounce (about 400 g) can black beans, drained but not rinsed

2 tablespoons barbecue sauce

½ cup (40 g) rolled oats (gluten-free, if necessary)

1. In a large bowl, mix all the ingredients.

2. Oil a skillet that has a lid.

3. Form the mixture into patties, using a scant ½ cup (100 g) of mixture for each patty.

4. Cook the patties over medium-high heat, covered with a lid, for 5 minutes.

5. Flip the patties—it's OK if they break up.

6. Cook the patties, uncovered, for another 2 to 3 minutes, breaking up the mixture into large chunks.

INTERNATIONAL YEAR OF PULSES

The United Nations General Assembly has declared 2016 International Year of Pulses. The UN states in its declaration that pulses (dried beans and peas) are "a vital source of plant-based proteins and amino acids for people around the globe and should be eaten as part of a healthy diet to address obesity, as well as to prevent and help manage chronic diseases such as diabetes, coronary conditions, and cancer . . . " Happily, pulses and grains are a great pair, so if you are looking for a way to celebrate the humble bean during its special year, consider giving some of these recipes a try:

• Millet and Poblano Chili (page 46)

• Multigrain Veggie Burger Crumbles (page 62)

• Chickpea Hemp Veggie Burgers (page 69)

You will appreciate the hearty textures, strong nutritional profiles, and delicious flavors that these ancient partners provide.

TEFF-LENTIL SLOPPY JOES

MAKES 4 SERVINGS

My family likes the tang of ketchup in these protein-rich sloppy joes, but they're just as delicious with crushed tomatoes. Either way, you're sure to love this old-school favorite made healthier with iron-rich lentils and nutty teff. These sloppy joes are delicious served over homemade Spelt Oat Bread (page 72) or Gluten-free Beer Bread (page 77). For a change of pace, serve Teff-Lentil Sloppy Joes over baked potatoes or baked sweet potatoes.

¼ cup (50 g) teff

1 cup (200 g) brown lentils

1 medium onion, diced

1 medium green bell pepper, ribs and seeds removed, diced

2 cloves garlic, minced

1 tablespoon olive oil

1¼ cups (300 g) ketchup or crushed tomatoes

1 tablespoon prepared yellow mustard

⅛ to ¼ teaspoon cayenne pepper

1. In a small pot, combine the teff with 1 cup (250 mL) water. Bring to a boil, reduce the heat, and simmer for 10 to 15 minutes, or until the water is absorbed and the grain is tender. Set aside.

2. Pick through the lentils and remove any stones or debris. Rinse. In a medium pot with a lid, combine the lentils with 4 cups (1 L) water. Bring to a boil, reduce the heat, and simmer, loosely covered with the lid, for 20 minutes, or until the lentils are tender. Drain any excess water.

3. In a large sauté pan, heat the oil over medium-high heat. Add the onion, green pepper, and garlic and sauté for 3 to 5 minutes, or until tender.

4. Add the teff and lentils to the pan. Mix in the ketchup or crushed tomatoes, mustard, and cayenne.

6. Heat through and serve.

MIGHTY TEFF

Teff is a crucial crop in Ethiopia, where it helps feed the second-most-populated country in Sub-Saharan Africa, thanks to its ability to withstand difficult growing conditions. While wheat grows best at 60°F, teff can thrive in temperatures close to 100°F, which is helpful in southern Ethiopia, where temperatures are frequently in the 80s and 90s. Teff also has a noteworthy yield. One pound of teff can produce up to one ton of teff in three months.

TEFF-BREADED EGGPLANT SLICES

MAKES 4 SERVINGS AS A SIDE DISH OR 2 SERVINGS AS A MAIN DISH

Tiny teff provides a nutrient-rich alternative to bread crumbs in this versatile dish that bakes up crunchy and flavorful. Serve the eggplant slices with Simplest Pasta Sauce (page 61) over A Quick and Easy Whole-Grain Pasta (page 67) or in a vegetarian sandwich. You can use teff to coat other veggies as well; I use this recipe to make teff-breaded zucchini and artichoke hearts, too. Once you start turning your vegetables into crunchy, flavorful treats, you won't want to stop! You can leave the skin on the eggplant or remove it. If you leave it on, the eggplant slices will be chewier.

Olive oil spray

1 eggplant

½ cup (100 g) teff

½ teaspoon garlic powder

¼ teaspoon salt

½ cup (120 mL) nondairy milk

1. Preheat the oven to 425°F (220°C/gas mark 7).

2. Line a baking sheet with parchment paper. Spray the parchment paper with olive oil.

3. With a sharp knife, cut the eggplant into ½-inch-thick slices.

4. In a shallow dish, combine the teff, garlic powder, and salt. Pour the nondairy milk into a shallow bowl.

5. Dip each slice of eggplant in the nondairy milk and then in the teff mixture.

6. Lay each slice on the prepared baking sheet. Spray with olive oil. Repeat with the remaining eggplant slices.

7. Bake for 50 minutes, or until the eggplant is crispy.

INJERA

If you've ever been to an Ethiopian restaurant, you've probably enjoyed injera, a flatbread made from teff. The batter is fermented, giving it a slightly sour taste. Stews or salads are served on top of the injera, allowing any liquids to soak into the porous bread. Bits of injera are torn off to scoop up stew, sauces, or salad, and then eaten. You can buy authentic injera, made in Ethiopia, in international or specialty markets.

FARRO AND CASHEW CREAM SAUCE

MAKES 4 SERVINGS

This take on macaroni and cheese has the same comforting creaminess as the traditional dish, and so much more. You'll be glad to serve this version made with ancient grains to your family instead of a commercial boxed version, which contains unhealthy additives. You can also substitute sorghum for farro if you need this dish to be gluten-free. Farro and Cashew Cream Sauce is a bit of a blank slate, so feel free to add some (or all) of the add-ins mentioned below to jazz up this dish.

¼ cup (40 g) cashews (Please see step one before beginning.)

½ cup (125 mL) water

2 tablespoons potato starch

1½ teaspoons olive oil

1 clove garlic

¼ teaspoon salt

1 teaspoon lemon juice

1 cup (240 mL) nondairy milk

1 tablespoon soy sauce

1 tablespoon nutritional yeast (optional)

4 cups (800 g) prepared farro (page 24) or sorghum (for a gluten-free option, page 22)

OPTIONAL ADD-INS
Steamed broccoli
Sautéed mushrooms
Green peas (fresh or frozen)
Giardiniera or other spicy vegetable mix

1. If you are using a high-power blender, you don't need to soak the cashews first, but if you have a standard blender, you will need to soak the cashews in water to cover for at least 2 hours before blending them. Drain and rinse the cashews before adding them to the blender.

2. In a blender, add the cashews, water, potato starch, olive oil, garlic, salt, and lemon juice and blend until smooth.

3. Pour the cashew mixture into a medium saucepan. Cook over medium heat, stirring, until the sauce thickens, approximately 3 to 4 minutes.

4. Add the nondairy milk, soy sauce, and nutritional yeast, if desired, to the sauce. Stir until well combined.

5. Remove the saucepan from the heat and mix the farro into the sauce. Stir in any desired add-ins.

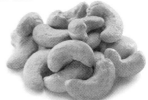

ARTICHOKE FARRO (OR SORGHUM)

MAKES 4 SERVINGS

I love fresh artichokes eaten all on their own, and I love frozen or canned artichoke hearts mixed into other dishes. This entrée highlights my beloved artichokes and really lets them shine. Farro has been enjoyed in Italy for thousands of years, so it's a natural partner for artichokes—another Italian favorite. I like to serve Artichoke Farro with ripe, sliced tomatoes on the side and a piece of Spelt Oat Bread (page 72) to sop up any extra liquid.

1   tablespoon olive oil

½   cup (80 g) diced onion

3   cloves garlic, minced

6   artichoke hearts (fresh, frozen and thawed, or canned), diced

¼   teaspoon salt

1   teaspoon dried thyme

1   teaspoon dried basil

1   teaspoon dried oregano

¼   teaspoon black pepper

2   tablespoons tomato paste

¼ to ½ teaspoon red pepper flakes (optional)

4   cups (800 g) prepared farro (or sorghum, a gluten-free option) (pages 24 and 22)

1. In a large skillet or sauté pan, heat the olive oil over medium heat.

2. Add onion and garlic and sauté for about 3 minutes, or until softened and fragrant.

3. Add the artichoke hearts, salt, thyme, basil, oregano, black pepper, tomato paste, and red pepper flakes, if desired, and cook, stirring until heated through.

4. Serve the farro (or sorghum) mixed with the artichoke hearts.

FOOD OF LEGIONS

Farro has been grown in Italy for thousands of years. It is believed that at the beginning of the common era, the Roman legions were fed rations of farro to keep them strong. That would not be surprising, given that farro is rich in fiber, protein, and vitamins and minerals, including niacin, magnesium, zinc, and iron. Although farro lost popularity over the years due to higher-yielding wheat varieties, its nutty flavor and firm texture have found a spot on menus at the finest restaurants across Italy and Europe and the United States over the past decade or two. Modern-day warriors (even if they're just the weekend tennis-playing variety) can now find farro at well-stocked grocery stores and health food shops to better fuel their adventures.

A QUICK AND EASY WHOLE-GRAIN PASTA

MAKES 2 GENEROUS SERVINGS

Have you ever wanted to try your hand at making your own pasta but felt intimidated by the equipment? This pasta couldn't be easier. No special equipment is needed, and it's fun to make because it's so hands-on. (Dinner guests—and your kids—will enjoy being involved in the process.) This pasta is firm, with a toothsome bite, and holds up well to a hearty tomato sauce with Multigrain Veggie Burger Crumbles (page 62) or Teff-breaded Eggplant Slices (page 64) served on top. This pasta comes together so quickly that it is practically ready in the time it takes the water to boil.

⅓ to ½ cup (80 to 120 mL) water

2 cups (240 g) whole-grain spelt flour, plus more as needed

1. Fill a large stockpot with water. Bring to a boil.

2. In a large, shallow bowl, mix ⅓ cup water into the flour a little at a time. Continue adding water, 1 tablespoon at a time, until the dough holds together but still seems relatively dry. (You may need up to ½ cup—120 mL—water.)

3. On a clean surface, knead the dough until smooth, about 5 minutes. If the dough sticks to the surface, sprinkle it with a little extra flour.

4. Form the dough into a ball. Divide it in half, then divide each half into four pieces.

5. Cover the dough with a damp towel.

6. Pinch off one piece of dough at a time and roll it into a snake, ½ inch (1 cm) thick and approximately 10 inches (25 cm) long. Cut each "snake" into ½-inch (1-cm) pieces.

7. Using your fingers, flatten each piece of dough into an oval. Indent each oval so that it's thinner in the middle than at the edges. The shape should resemble orichette.

8. Place the pasta on a large plate or platter.

9. Repeat the same process with the remaining pieces of dough.

10. When all the dough has been prepared, drop the pieces into the boiling water.

11. Boil until the pasta floats to the top, about 4 minutes.

12. Remove with a slotted spoon. Serve with your favorite pasta sauce.

HUMMUS ARUGULA FLATBREAD

4 SERVINGS

This recipe is just one example of how a flatbread can easily be transformed into a light, nutritious meal with layers of flavor. Here, hummus, a protein- and iron-rich spread, beautifully balances the nuttiness of the flatbread and complements the peppery zing of arugula, creating a symphony of flavors in each bite. Pair this sandwich with a cup of hearty Creamy Potato Millet Soup (page 45) and you have a satisfying meal.

¼ cup (200 g) *Lemon Artichoke Hummus (recipe follows)*

4 *Spelt Flatbreads (page 76)*

1 *medium tomato, sliced*

¼ cup (5 g) *arugula*

Squeeze of lemon juice

1. Spread the hummus on each flatbread, dividing equally.

2. Top with the tomato and arugula.

3. Add a squeeze of lemon juice over the top of each flatbread.

LEMON ARTICHOKE HUMMUS

MAKES 2 CUPS

1 *15-ounce (about 400 g) can cannellini beans, drained and rinsed*

1 *15-ounce (about 400 g) can artichoke hearts, drained and rinsed*

1 *large clove garlic*

Zest and juice of 1 or 2 lemons to taste

¼ *teaspoon salt*

1. In a food processor or blender, puree all the ingredients together.

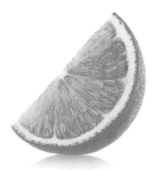

CHAPTER 7

BAKED GOODS

While it's convenient to pick up a loaf of bread or a box of donuts at the grocery store, it's much more soul-satisfying, not to mention nourishing, to whip up your own baked goods at home. Working with ancient grains brings a whole new level of wholesomeness to your baking.

Whole-grain spelt is a dream to bake with. You get all of the health benefits of baking with a whole grain—specifically minerals like iron, manganese, phosphorus, magnesium, and zinc, all of which contribute to strong bones and healthy blood and immune systems. Spelt is also a good source of protein and fiber, so eating a sandwich made with Spelt Sandwich Loaf (page 73) will keep you energized and feeling sated over several hours. But the benefits of baking with spelt extend beyond its exemplary health profile. Spelt bakes up into a nutty, full-flavored whole-grain loaf that's still light in texture. In fact, spelt adds texture and flavor to all of your favorite treats, from cookies to brownies to cakes.

Other ancient grains also contribute to baked goods that are not only better for you, but taste great. Oat flour is slightly sweet and has a higher moisture content than other flours, making for tender Chocolate Chip Scones (page 74) and moist Peach Mango Muffins (page 82). Teff and sorghum add protein and depth of flavor to gluten-free baked goods like Multigrain Gluten-free Biscuits (page 79).

Once you experience the full flavors, lovely textures, and health benefits of baking with ancient grains, you will want to keep them stocked in your pantry or refrigerator.

BIBLICAL GRAINS

Ancient grains—wheat, barley, spelt, rye, and oats—are mentioned in the Bible, particularly in Exodus, which tells the story of the Israelites' hasty departure from Egypt. It was so hasty that they could not wait for their dough to rise. The result was matzoh, which is eaten every year during Passover to commemorate the Exodus. Some Jewish scholars believe that the unleavened bread was made from spelt.

OPPOSITE: **Chocolate Chip Scones, page 74**

SPELT OAT BREAD

MAKES 1 LOAF

This rustic loaf combines a touch of sweetness from maple syrup and a pleasant chewiness from the oats. It is equally delicious fresh from the oven or toasted a couple of days later. If you aren't going to eat the whole loaf at once, though, let it cool completely before slicing it.

- 1½ cups (350 mL) lukewarm water
- 1 packet (1½ tablespoons, or 21 g) active dry yeast
- 2 teaspoons salt
- 1½ tablespoons maple syrup
- 1½ tablespoons olive oil, plus more for greasing the pan
- 4 cups (500 g) whole-grain spelt flour
- 1 cup (80 g) rolled oats

1. In a large bowl, combine the water, yeast, salt, maple syrup, and olive oil.

2. Add the flour and oats and thoroughly mix together.

3. Loosely cover the bowl with a lid or a kitchen towel and let the dough rise for 2 hours (or more) in a warm room. If your room is cooler, you might need to let the dough rise longer. Once risen, it should be about twice the original volume.

4. Preheat the oven to 425°F (220°C/gas mark 7).

5. Lightly coat a loaf pan with olive oil. Transfer the risen dough into the oiled pan.

6. Bake for 40 minutes, or until the bread is golden brown.

7. Remove the bread from the pan and cool on a rack. Cool completely before slicing.

TO SLICE OR NOT TO SLICE

One of life's great pleasures is fresh-baked bread. I love the way the fragrance of baking bread fills my home. I wait in anticipation for the golden loaf to come out of the oven. It takes all of my willpower not to slice off a big chunk while it's still piping hot and eat it right then and there. Why wait? Why not enjoy all of that crusty, steamy, soft-centered goodness straight from the oven? The truth is, your bread will be much improved if you let it rest for a while (unless, of course, you plan on eating the whole loaf right away). Here's why: When you slice into hot bread, all the steam that keeps it moist escapes. If you wait for the bread to cool, you won't lose any steam when you slice it, and it will retain enough moisture to keep from drying out. If I plan to serve a loaf of freshly baked bread with soup for dinner, however, and I know my family will eat it right away, I don't need to wait, but if the bread will be used for sandwiches throughout the week, I resist temptation and wait for it to cool.

SPELT SANDWICH LOAF

MAKES 1 LOAF

One of the qualities that I love about baking with spelt is how it reacts with yeast. I used to be afraid of baking yeast loaves. All of the kneading and waiting, and then more kneading, are too much for me. Whole-grain spelt flour, however, rises with lots of lovely air pockets after it is mixed with yeast, water, and a little salt. All you have to do is wait for the first rise, and the dough is ready to bake. You can form the dough into a round shape or transfer the dough into a loaf pan to make a standard loaf. Either way, you will get a tender crust if you brush the top of the loaf with water before baking. Skip this step, however, if you want a sturdier crust.

1½ cups (350 mL) lukewarm water

¼ ounce (2¼ teaspoons, or 7 g) active dry yeast

1 teaspoon salt

3¼ cups (400 g) whole-grain spelt flour, plus more for dusting

Olive oil, for coating the pan

1. In a large bowl, combine the water, yeast, and salt.

2. Add the flour and stir until just mixed; do not overmix.

3. Loosely cover the bowl with a lid or a kitchen towel and let the dough rise for 2 hours (or more) in a warm room. If your room is cooler, you might need to let the dough rise longer. Once risen, it should be about twice the original volume.

4. Preheat the oven to 425°F (220°C/gas mark 7).

5. Lightly coat a standard loaf pan with olive oil.

6. Dust the risen dough with a little more flour. Loosely shape the dough into a football shape.

7. Place the dough in the oiled pan. Brush the top of the bread lightly with water before baking if you want a more tender crust.

8. Bake for 35 to 40 minutes, or until the top is golden brown and the loaf makes a hollow sound when you give it a gentle knock on the bottom.

9. Remove the bread from the pan and cool on a rack. Cool completely before slicing.

CHOCOLATE CHIP SCONES

MAKES 8 SCONES

Scones are one of my favorite baked goods. These come together quickly and are delicious on their own or spread with some raspberry preserves. These scones use nondairy yogurt for moisture in place of shortening or butter, making them a treat that you can indulge in and still feel good about. If you grind your own oat flour for these scones, the texture will be a little more like a granola bar, but they'll still be very tasty.

- 2 cups (200 g) oat flour, plus more for dusting (gluten-free, if necessary)
- ⅓ cup (50 g) evaporated cane juice or coconut palm sugar
- 1 tablespoon baking powder
- ½ teaspoon salt
- 1 teaspoon vanilla extract
- 1 6-ounce (170 g) container nondairy yogurt (vanilla or coconut flavored, or plain)
- ½ cup (100 g) chocolate chips

1. Preheat the oven to 350°F (180°C/gas mark 4). Line a baking sheet with parchment paper.

2. In a large bowl, whisk together the flour, sugar, baking powder, and salt.

3. Mix the vanilla into the yogurt.

4. Stir the yogurt mixture into the flour mixture. Stir the chocolate chips into the dough.

5. Shape the dough into a flattened disk, about 6 inches across.

6. Cut the disk into 8 wedges. Place the wedges on the parchment-lined baking sheet.

7. Bake for 12 to 14 minutes, until the scones are puffed and golden.

OAT-LOVING PUPS

Not all people food is safe for dogs. Oats, however, are not only safe for our canine friends, but can be good for them, too. Dogs can benefit from the same anti-itch properties that make oats soothing to itchy human skin. Mix up an oat bath with ¼ cup (2 g) ground oats in a bath filled partway with tepid water) and let your dog rest in it. If your pup is not a fan of baths, you can saturate a washcloth in the oat-soaked water and place it on any itchy areas. You can also feed your dog cooked oatmeal mixed in with the food. A tablespoon or two of cooked oatmeal can really help keep your dog's digestion working well.

BLUEBERRY SCONES

MAKES 8 SCONES

These delicious scones bring ancient grains to teatime. Blueberry yogurt makes them fragrant, and the little bursts of whole blueberries scattered throughout keep the scones moist. Is there anything better than curling up with a good book while snacking on a blueberry scone and a cup of hot tea?

2 cups (240 g) whole-grain spelt flour

2 teaspoons baking powder

½ teaspoon salt

1 6-ounce (170 g) container blueberry nondairy yogurt

½ cup (120 mL) nondairy milk

½ cup (75 g) blueberries, fresh or frozen

2 teaspoons evaporated cane juice or coconut palm sugar

1. Preheat the oven to 400°F (200°C/gas mark 6). Line a baking sheet with parchment paper.

2. In a medium bowl, whisk together the flour, baking powder, and salt.

3. Mix in the yogurt and nondairy milk. Mix in the blueberries.

4. Shape the dough into a flattened disk, about 6 inches across.

5. Cut the disk into 8 wedges. Place the wedges on the parchment-lined baking sheet.

6. Sprinkle a little sugar on top of each wedge, dividing evenly.

7. Bake for 12 to 14 minutes, until the scones are puffed and golden.

SPELT TORTILLAS OR FLATBREADS

MAKES 16 TORTILLAS OR FLATBREADS

If you roll this dough very thin, you will make lovely tortillas, and if you roll it out a little less, the result will be a little thicker, sturdier flatbread. Either way, they are delicious. For soft-shell tacos, spoon some Millet and Poblano Chili (page 46) or Sorghum Taco filling (page 55) into a tortilla and top it with avocado, lettuce, and tomatoes. Or, to turn these flatbreads into croutons or crackers, just toast them after they cool. You can enjoy leftover tortillas or flatbreads one or two days later, simply by reheating them.

- 3 cups (360 g) whole-grain spelt flour, plus more for dusting
- 1 teaspoon salt
- 1 teaspoon baking powder
- ⅓ cup (70 mL) neutral oil (sunflower, grape-seed, or canola)
- 1 cup (250 mL) water

1. In a food processor (you can also use a stand mixer fitted with a dough hook), pulse the flour, salt, and baking powder together 3 times to combine.

2. Add the oil and water and process for 1 minute.

3. Remove the resulting dough from the food processor. Dust the dough in whole-grain spelt flour, place it in a large bowl covered with a clean dish towel, and let it rest at room temperature for 5 to 10 minutes.

4. Divide the dough into 16 equal-size balls. Roll out each ball into a thin disk about 5 inches (13 cm) in diameter. For tortillas, roll out the dough very thinly; for flatbreads, leave them a little thicker.

5. Heat a dry skillet or griddle over medium-high heat.

6. Cook each tortilla or flatbread for about 2 minutes, until it is golden on one side. Flip and cook it on the other side until it has a nice golden color.

7. Stack the tortillas on top of one another until you are ready to serve them.

8. Extra tortillas can be wrapped tightly in wax paper and aluminum foil and stored in the refrigerator for up to 3 days. Reheat the tortillas in a dry skillet or toaster.

GLUTEN-FREE BEER BREAD

MAKES 1 LOAF

Thankfully, gluten-free beer is now readily available almost everywhere. In this recipe, gluten-free beer takes the place of dry yeast, making it easy to create bread with a great texture that is perfect for toasting, spreading with hummus, or eating warm from the oven. Much of the alcohol will bake out of the bread, but enough will remain to give it a distinctive, beery flavor.

1   tablespoon plus 1 teaspoon olive oil

2½ cups (225 g) oat flour

½ cup (60 g) sweet white sorghum flour

1½ teaspoons salt

1½ teaspoons baking powder

¼ cup (35 g) evaporated cane juice or coconut palm sugar

12 ounces (350 mL) gluten-free beer

1. Preheat the oven to 375°F (190°C/gas mark 5).

2. Lightly oil a standard loaf pan with 1 teaspoon of olive oil.

3. In a medium bowl, whisk together the flours, salt, baking powder, and sugar.

4. In a medium bowl, combine the remaining 1 tablespoon olive oil and beer.

5. Add the beer mixture to the flour mixture. Stir well.

6. Transfer the batter into the oiled pan.

7. Bake for 45 to 50 minutes, or until the bread is golden brown.

8. Run a knife around the perimeter of the pan. Let the bread cool in the pan for 10 minutes.

9. After 10 minutes, remove the bread from the pan and let it cool completely on a cooling rack before cutting.

CHEERS! ANCIENT GRAINS BRING THE BREW BACK TO GLUTEN-FREE BEER DRINKERS

Beer is traditionally made from barley, hops, yeast, and water—ingredients that make a wide range of flavorful brews. If you need to follow a gluten-free diet, however, gluten-rich barley is not a guest you want at your party. Fortunately, creative brewers have turned to ancient grains, like sorghum and millet, to stand in for barley and to produce high-quality beers that happen to be gluten-free. These delicious beers come in a wide range of styles, from traditional ales to saisons to stouts. Thanks to ancient grains, every beer drinker can find the perfect brew.

GARLIC FLATBREAD

MAKES 16 FLATBREADS

The crispiness or chewiness of this wonderful, garlicky flatbread depends on how thin you roll the dough. If you want a more cracker-like result, roll out the dough into a thin disk that is greater than five inches (13 cm) in diameter. Adding herbs or other aromatics, like oregano or shallots, to the oil, in place of the garlic, will give you a flatbread with a different flavor. Don't be shy about experimenting with your favorite flavorings. Serve Garlic Flatbread alongside a bowl of A Quick and Easy Whole-Grain Pasta (page 67) with red sauce and Multigrain Veggie Burger Crumbles (page 62).

- *3 cups (360 g) whole-grain spelt flour, plus more for dusting*
- *1 teaspoon salt*
- *1 teaspoon baking powder*
- *1 cup (250 mL) water*
- *½ cup (120 mL) olive oil, divided*
- *2 cloves garlic, minced*

1. Preheat the oven to 425°F (220°C/gas mark 7).

2. In a food processor, pulse together the flour, salt, and baking powder.

3. Add the water and ¼ cup (60 mL) olive oil. Process for 1 minute.

4. Remove from the food processor and form the dough into a ball. Dust it with extra flour and set it aside.

5. In a small saucepan, add the minced garlic to ¼ cup (60 mL) olive oil and heat until the garlic is fragrant. Set aside.

6. Line 2 baking sheets with parchment paper.

7. Divide the dough into 16 equal-size balls. Roll out each ball into a thin disk, about 5 inches (13 cm) in diameter. For crisper flatbreads, roll out the dough very thinly; for chewier flatbreads, leave them a little thicker.

8. Place each flatbread on a parchment-lined baking sheet. Brush each flatbread with the garlic-infused oil.

9. Bake for 10 minutes, or until the breads are lightly golden.

MULTIGRAIN GLUTEN-FREE BISCUITS

MAKES 10 BISCUITS

Teff and sorghum are combined with brown rice flour in these tender, slightly sweet, and nutty biscuits. Unlike other multigrain breads, these biscuits are light and fluffy. The flaxseed meal and soured nondairy milk bind the flours without xanthan or guar gum. These biscuits can turn a simple bowl of soup or plate of salad into a robust meal.

FLEXIBLE FLATBREAD

What if just one recipe could be the star of many delicious meals? Flatbread is that versatile player, and here are just a few of the roles it can play at mealtime:

- Fill flatbread with chili and top with shredded lettuce, diced onions, and cilantro for a quick taco.
- Spread flatbread with pesto and sliced tomatoes for an elegant appetizer.
- Use flatbread as the base for a make-your-own-pizza night.
- Make flatbread croutons and cut them into cracker-size pieces to accompany your favorite dip.
- Spread hummus on flatbread, then load on veggies—thinly sliced carrots, radishes, tomatoes, and sprouts, etc.—for an out-of-this-world veggie sandwich.
- Serve flatbread alongside a bowl of soup for a light meal.
- Spread flatbread with almond butter and top with sliced strawberries for a filling and delicious breakfast sandwich.

---

1 cup (240 mL) nondairy milk

1 teaspoon lemon juice

2 tablespoons flaxseed meal

½ cup (90 g) teff flour (or if teff flour is not available in your market, teff grain ground into a flour in a clean coffee grinder)

1¼ cup (200 g) brown rice flour

¼ cup (30 g) sweet white sorghum flour

1 teaspoon baking powder

½ teaspoon baking soda

¼ cup (100 g) non-hydrogenated vegetable shortening

1. Preheat the oven to 425°F (220°C/gas mark 7). Line a baking sheet with parchment paper.

2. In a small bowl, stir the lemon juice into the nondairy milk. Stir in the flaxseed meal and set aside.

3. In a large bowl, whisk together the flours, baking powder, and baking soda.

4. Cut the shortening into the flour mixture using a pastry cutter or two knives. Stir in the nondairy milk mixture and combine thoroughly.

5. Drop the batter by the ¼ cup (about 150 g) onto the parchment-lined baking sheet.

6. Bake for 15 minutes, or until the biscuits are golden brown. Enjoy warm from the oven or cooled to room temperature.

TENDER CORNBREAD

MAKES 9 PIECES

You won't believe that this light and fluffy cornbread is made with whole grains, but it is. And if you use vanilla nondairy yogurt in the mix, the flavor of the cornbread will be lightly sweet. Try it for breakfast with your favorite preserves, or bake it with plain yogurt for a more savory bread to serve with a bowl of Tomato Soup (page 46) for a light lunch.

- 3 *tablespoons neutral oil (sunflower, grape-seed, or canola) plus extra for oiling the pan*
- 1 *cup (120 g) cornmeal*
- 1 *cup (120 g) whole-grain spelt flour*
- ¼ *cup (35 g) evaporated cane juice or coconut palm sugar*
- 2 *teaspoons baking powder*
- 1 *teaspoon baking soda*
- ½ *teaspoon salt*
- ¼ *cup (65 g) applesauce*
- 1 *cup (240 mL) nondairy milk*
- ½ *cup (120 g) nondairy yogurt (plain or vanilla)*

1. Preheat the oven to 400°F (200°C/gas mark 6). Lightly oil an 8- or 9-inch-square (20- or 23-cm) baking pan.

2. In a medium bowl, whisk together the cornmeal, flour, sugar, baking powder, baking soda, and salt.

3. In a large bowl, mix together the applesauce, nondairy milk, nondairy yogurt, and oil.

4. Mix the dry ingredients into the wet ingredients.

5. Spread the batter into the prepared baking pan.

6. Bake for 20 to 25 minutes, or until a toothpick inserted into the center of the cornbread comes out clean.

THE GLUTEN-FARRO-SPELT DYNAMIC

Both farro and spelt are the result of the earliest form of wheat (einkorn) cross-pollinating with other grasses. Their protein structure is different from modern wheat's, which means that their gluten is different from the gluten in modern wheat. Interestingly, some people who are gluten intolerant can eat farro and spelt without the gastrointestinal distress they experience after eating modern wheat. People who have celiac disease, a wheat allergy, or another medically diagnosed gluten intolerance, however, should avoid eating farro and spelt unless a doctor has advised otherwise.

SAVORY DROP BISCUITS

MAKES 4–7 BISCUITS

These drop biscuits are full of flavor. You can make them larger (a yield of 4 biscuits) and slice them in half for sandwiches—using them with the Chickpea Hemp Veggie Burgers (page 69) makes a particularly tasty combo—or you can keep them on the small side (a yield of 4 to 7 biscuits) and serve them with soup or salad to bring an extra boost of flavor to your meal. They are really special served with Creamy Potato Millet Soup (page 45).

- *1 cup (240 mL) nondairy milk*
- *1 teaspoon apple cider vinegar*
- *1¾ cups (210 g) whole-grain spelt flour*
- *1 teaspoon baking powder*
- *½ teaspoon baking soda*
- *¼ teaspoon smoked paprika*
- *¼ teaspoon ground cumin*
- *⅛ teaspoon garlic powder*
- *¼ cup (50 g) non-hydrogenated vegetable shortening*

1. Preheat the oven to 425°F (220°C/gas mark 7).

2. In a cup, combine the nondairy milk with the apple cider vinegar. Set aside.

NUTRIENT-RICH GLUTEN-FREE FLOUR BLENDS

With the increase in the number of people who are now following a gluten-free diet, a plethora of gluten-free flour blends are available at well-stocked grocery stores. Many gluten-free flour blends, however, are made with nutrient-void starches and processed grains, so it really pays to look at the ingredient list before you buy. Flour blends that are rich in sorghum, millet, or teff (and without starches and processed grains) will have a richer nutrient profile, as well as taste better.

3. In a medium bowl, whisk together the flour, baking powder, baking soda, smoked paprika, cumin, and garlic powder.

4. Cut the shortening into the flour mixture with a pastry cutter or two knives. Stir in the nondairy milk mixture and combine thoroughly.

5. Drop the batter by the ¼ cup (about 150 g) onto a parchment-lined baking sheet.

6. Bake for 12 to 15 minutes, or until the biscuits are golden brown and fragrant.

7. Remove the biscuits to a cooling rack, or eat them warm.

PEACH MANGO MUFFINS

MAKES 12 MUFFINS

These muffins are bursting with chunks of juicy fruit. They never last more than one day at my house, but if you have some that make it to the next day, they will taste best if you reheat them. Whether you serve Peach Mango Muffins with a special breakfast or enjoy them as an afternoon pick-me-up, they are always delicious. They are sweet enough to eat as a dessert, too.

2   *cups (200 g) oat flour (gluten-free, if necessary)*

1½ *teaspoons baking powder, divided*

½   *teaspoon salt*

½   *cup (125 g) applesauce*

½   *cup (110 mL) neutral oil (sunflower, grape-seed, or canola), plus more for oiling if needed*

¾   *cup (100 g) evaporated cane juice or coconut palm sugar*

¼   *cup (60 mL) nondairy milk*

1   *teaspoon vanilla extract*

1   *cup (250 g) peaches, small dice*

½   *cup (100 g) mango, small dice*

1. Preheat the oven to 350°F (175°C/gas mark 4). Line a standard muffin pan with paper liners or lightly oil the cups.

2. In a medium bowl, whisk together the flour, 1 teaspoon baking powder, and salt.

3. In a larger bowl, combine the applesauce, ½ teaspoon baking powder, oil, sugar, nondairy milk, and vanilla.

4. Stir the flour mixture into the applesauce mixture. Mix in the peaches and mangoes.

5. Divide the batter among the cups in the muffin pan.

6. Bake for 25 to 30 minutes, or until a toothpick inserted into the center of a muffin comes out clean.

7. Remove muffins to a cooling rack.

8. Although the muffins are very tender when they are first out of the oven, they will firm up as they cool.

GOOD FOOD ON THE ROAD

It's all too easy en route to stop at a fast-food restaurant or gas station for a quick meal or snack. But with a little planning, you can eat well in transit. Pack some Nutty Granola (page 39), Peach Mango Muffins (this page), or Cocoa Power Bites (page 40) and snack on healthy whole grains. Sandwiches on Spelt Sandwich Loaf (page 73) travel well, too, and with Whole Grain Chocolate Brownies (page 94), you can satisfy cravings with healthy treats.

RASPBERRY CHOCOLATE CHIP CAKE

MAKES 18 SERVINGS

This is what I like to call a snack cake. It's the kind of cake that you can make on a weeknight and serve after dinner. It's not over the top; it's just right. It has a lovely texture, and the fruit and chocolate add moisture and flavor and make frosting unnecessary. You can wrap and freeze individual pieces to enjoy on another day when you need a little treat.

- 1¾ cups (210 g) whole-grain spelt flour
- 1 cup (150 g) evaporated cane juice or coconut palm sugar
- 1 teaspoon baking soda
- ½ teaspoon salt
- 2 teaspoons vanilla extract
- ¼ cup (60 mL) neutral oil (sunflower, grape-seed, or canola)
- 1 cup (250 mL) water
- 2 teaspoons apple cider vinegar
- 1 cup (125 g) raspberries
- ½ cup (100 g) chocolate chips

1. Preheat the oven to 350°F (175°C/gas mark 4). Line the bottom of a 9 × 13-inch (23 × 33-cm) baking pan with parchment paper.

2. In a medium bowl, whisk together the flour, sugar, baking soda, and salt.

3. In a small bowl or measuring cup, mix the vanilla, oil, and water.

4. Stir the wet ingredients into the dry ones.

5. Stir the apple cider vinegar into the batter. Gently mix in the raspberries and chocolate chips.

6. Pour the batter into the parchment-lined baking pan.

HEALTH BENEFITS OF CHOCOLATE

Chocolate lovers have long known that chocolate makes you feel good. But chocolate isn't just good for the soul, it's also good for the body. Cocoa, and dark chocolate made from cocoa beans, is rich in flavonoids, compounds that act as antioxidants and prevent free radicals (which can be the products of exposure to environmental contaminants like cigarette smoke or pollution) from damaging cells in the body. Chocolate has also been shown to lower blood pressure and prevent LDL (bad cholesterol) from forming plaque in our arteries. To get these health benefits, though, it's best to choose dark chocolate that's at least 70 percent cocoa. The simpler the ingredient list, the better. It's nice to know that a little chocolate in moderation can be a very good thing.

SUSTAINABLITY AND ENVIRONMENTAL ISSUES

BIODEGRADABLE PACKING PEANUTS

Are you looking for a way to protect your shipments without hurting the environment? Ancient grains to the rescue! Many bio-degradable packing peanuts are made from sorghum starch. Unlike packing peanuts made from Styrofoam, ones made from sorghum don't have to go into a landfill after you open your package. Instead, they dissolve when exposed to water. Also, packing peanuts made from sorghum won't hurt your pet if he accidentally eats one. Biodegradable packing peanuts are just one more way that ancient grains are good for the planet.

SUSTAINABLE PALM OIL

Many of the products that we consume contain palm oil from the fruit of palm trees that grow primarily in Indonesia and Malaysia. There is great demand for this flavorless oil worldwide—not just for cooking, but also for use in shampoo, soap, and cosmetics, to name just a few of its applications. As a result, millions of tons of palm oil are produced and consumed each year. This demand, however, has led to some significant problems, including deforestation: Acres and acres of primary rain forest have been cleared for palm oil plantations, and native people have been removed from their land to make room for further expansion of this industry. When the rain forest is destroyed, the homes of many plants and animals are eliminated, as well.

But producing an alternative that isn't damaging to the environment, indigenous populations, or wildlife isn't as easy as just switching to another vegetable oil, mainly because of one very "good" economic reason to keep the industry alive and well: Palm is very efficient to grow. Other plants that produce oil require twice as much land for a comparable amount of oil.

Since 2004, industry representatives, NGOs that advocate for the environment and indigenous groups, and consumer product companies have come together in order to address these issues. For example, the Roundtable on Sustainable Palm Oil (RSPO) (www.rspo.org) certifies palm oil that is produced sustainably and focuses on protecting virgin forests, preventing the relocation of indigenous populations, defending workers' rights, and minimizing the use of pesticides.

Because palm oil stays creamy at room temperature and melts well, it can be an ally in the kitchen. I use palm-oil based non-hydrogenated vegetable shortening—from companies with a firm commitment to sustainable palm oil.

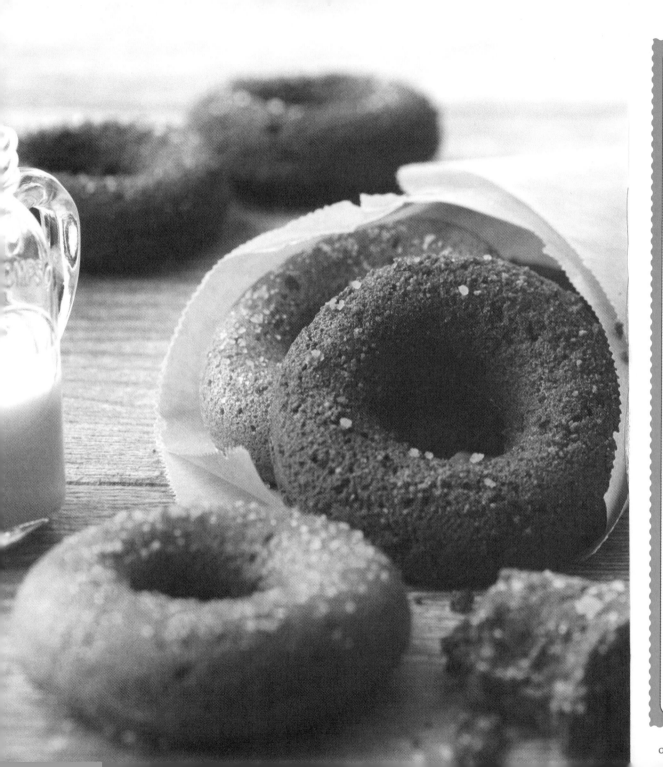

CHAPTER 8

DESSERTS

My family is most definitely a dessert family, and we have a sweet treat most evenings after dinner. When you indulge your sweet tooth as regularly as we do, it's important that your desserts bring something more than just a little sweetness to the plate. When ancient grains take center stage you can feel a little better about that indulgence.

Whether your choice of something sweet is fruity, like Pineapple Upside-Down Cake (page 91), or chocolaty, like Whole-Grain Chocolate Brownies (page 94), you get a nice serving of vitamins, minerals, protein, and fiber when you use oat, sorghum, or spelt flour.

In this chapter, oats make a surprising appearance in ice creams, too. I love the creaminess that oats bring to frozen desserts, and their natural sweetness marries well with other flavors in icy treats.

Millet makes an ideal whole-grain substitute for white rice in grain puddings. I think warm Coconut Millet Pudding (page 93) is the ultimate comfort food.

You never have to deny yourself a little treat if it includes nutrient-dense whole grains!

NUT-FREE OPTIONS

In the United States, eight foods—milk, eggs, tree nuts, peanuts, soy, wheat, fish, and shellfish—account for over 90 percent of all food allergies. Researchers from FARE (Food Allergy Research & Education), an organization that works on behalf of the millions of Americans who have food allergies, estimate that 1 in every 13 children (under the age of 18) has a food allergy. Not surprisingly, more and more schools and social settings where there are children are going "nut-free." Fortunately, seeds are a wonderful substitute. Use sunflower seed butter in place of peanut butter or almond butter, and your kids can enjoy many more of their favorite treats without worry. You can also use hemp seeds, sunflower seeds, or shelled pumpkin seeds (also known as pepitas) in place of almonds, pecans, walnuts, or cashews. And use oat milk (page 27) in place of almond milk or soy milk.

OPPOSITE: **Chocolate Donuts, page 96, and Pumpkin Donuts, page 97**

7. Bake for 30 to 35 minutes, or until a toothpick inserted into the center of the cake comes out clean. (You might see some melted chocolate, but there should be no batter.)

8. Let the cake cool in the pan, set on a cooling rack, for 10 minutes.

9. Remove the cake from the pan and set on the rack to cool completely.

CHOCOLATE OAT CAKE

MAKES 9 SERVINGS

I love chocolate cakes—and recipes for it, whether for light, cocoa-flavored cakes or richer, denser, darker cakes. Chocolate Oat Cake is definitely a richer one! Moist and densely chocolaty, it can be served in small pieces on its own or topped with ice cream or sorbet. Olive oil may seem like a strange ingredient, but the fruity oil complements the chocolate. amazingly well.

1¼ cups (125 g) oat flour (gluten-free, if necessary)

¼ cup (30 g) sweet white sorghum flour

⅓ cup (30 g) cocoa powder

1 teaspoon baking soda

½ teaspoon salt

1 cup (150 g) evaporated cane juice or coconut palm sugar

½ cup (120 mL) olive oil

1 cup (250 mL) brewed coffee

1 tablespoon vanilla extract

1 tablespoon apple cider vinegar

½ cup (100 g) chocolate chips

1. Preheat the oven to 375°F (190°C/gas mark 5). Line an 8- or 9-inch square (20- or 23-cm) baking pan with parchment paper.

2. In a medium bowl, whisk together the flours, cocoa powder, baking soda, salt, and sugar.

3. In a smaller bowl or measuring cup, mix the oil, coffee, and vanilla extract.

4. Pour the oil mixture into the flour mixture and combine well.

5. Stir in the apple cider vinegar. Stir in the chocolate chips.

6. Pour the batter into the parchment-lined pan.

7. Bake for 30 to 35 minutes, or until a toothpick inserted into the center of the cake comes out clean. (You might see some melted chocolate, but there should be no batter.)

8. Let the cake cool in the pan, set on a cooling rack, for 10 minutes.

9. Remove the cake from the pan and set on the rack to cool completely.

CHOCOLATE ZUCCHINI CAKE

MAKES 20 SERVINGS

This snack cake relies on zucchini for its moist texture and provides many important nutrients that your body needs, including copper, vitamin C, and magnesium. Chocolate Zucchini Cake is a good option for bake sales, because the chocolate chips and zucchini help keep individual slices from drying out.

¼ cup (60 mL) neutral oil (sunflower, grape-seed, or canola), plus more for oiling

2¾ cups (275 g) oat flour (gluten-free, if necessary)

1 teaspoon baking soda

1¾ teaspoons baking powder, divided

½ cup (50 g) cocoa powder

1 teaspoon salt

¾ cup (200 g) applesauce

½ cup (160 mL) maple syrup

½ cup (75 g) evaporated cane juice or coconut palm sugar

½ cup flaxseed meal

1 tablespoon vanilla extract

2 cups (350 g) grated zucchini

1 cup (175 g) chocolate chips

1. Preheat the oven to 350°F (180°C/gas mark 4). Lightly oil a 9 × 13-inch (23 × 33-cm) baking pan.

2. In a medium bowl, whisk together the flour, baking soda, 1 teaspoon baking powder, cocoa, and salt.

3. In a large bowl, combine the applesauce with the remaining ¾ teaspoon baking powder.

4. Add the ¼ cup oil, maple syrup, sugar, flaxseed meal, and vanilla to the applesauce mixture. Combine.

5. Add the flour mixture to the applesauce mixture and combine.

6. Stir in the zucchini and chocolate chips until well combined.

7. Pour the batter into the oiled pan.

8. Bake for 25 minutes, or until a toothpick inserted in the center of the cake comes out clean. Cool on a cooling rack.

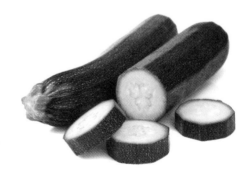

PEANUT BUTTER SNACK CAKE

MAKES 24 SERVINGS

If you want this snack cake to be nut-free you can substitute the peanut butter with sunflower seed butter. Don't be alarmed, though, if it turns a little green while baking. Sunflower seeds can have a chemical reaction with alkaline substances like baking soda, which gives this cake a slightly greenish cast. It's still safe to eat and quite delicious.

- 1 tablespoon neutral oil (sunflower, grape-seed, or canola), for oiling the pan
- 1¾ cups (210 g) whole-grain spelt flour (oat flour if you need this cake to be gluten-free)
- 1 teaspoon baking powder
- ½ teaspoon baking soda
- ¼ teaspoon salt
- 1 cup (250 g) applesauce
- ¾ cup (235 mL) maple syrup
- 1 cup (250 g) peanut butter (crunchy or smooth)
- ¾ cup (130 g) chocolate chips (optional)

1. Preheat the oven to 375°F (190°C/gas mark 5).

2. Oil a 9 × 13-inch (22 × 33-cm) baking pan or line it with parchment paper.

3. In a medium bowl, whisk together the flour, baking powder, baking soda, and salt.

4. In a large bowl, mix the applesauce, maple syrup, and peanut butter.

5. Stir the flour mixture into the applesauce mixture.

6. Pour the batter into the prepared pan.

7. Bake for 18 to 20 minutes, or until a toothpick inserted into the center of the cake comes out clean. To serve, cut the cake into individual squares, as you would for brownies.

MAPLE SYRUP GETS BETTER GRADES

Until recently, several grades of maple syrup were available to consumers, including Fancy, Grade A, and Grade B. Grade C was available commercially. In 2014, Vermont led the way in renaming them. The different grades were always identical in quality, and the letters were based on color and strength of maple flavor. All syrup is now Grade A, and the new names describe the differences in flavor: Golden Color and Delicate Taste; Amber Color and Rich Flavor; Dark Color and Robust Flavor; Very Dark Color and Strong Flavor. I have always preferred the darker color and richer maple flavor of Grade B, whether for topping pancakes or sweetening baked goods. Grade A: Dark Color and Robust Flavor matches up most closely with the former Grade B.

LEMON COCONUT-OIL POUND CAKE

MAKES 8 SERVINGS

This simple and elegant cake is a dinner-party-worthy dessert, especially when it's dressed up with a little glaze. The warm flavor of the spelt flour also blends in seamlessly with the tart lemon and smooth coconut oil to make a lovely crumb. Serve this wonderful pound cake with some fresh raspberries for a really beautiful presentation.

FOR THE CAKE
2   teaspoons lemon zest
1   cup (150 g) evaporated cane juice or coconut palm sugar
½   cup (110 g) coconut oil, soft but firm, plus more for oiling pan
1   cup (250 g) applesauce
2   tablespoons lemon juice
1½ cups (180 g) whole-grain spelt flour
1   teaspoon baking powder
¼   teaspoon baking soda
½   teaspoon salt

FOR THE GLAZE (OPTIONAL)
2   tablespoons powdered sugar
2   teaspoons lemon juice

MAKE THE CAKE

1. Preheat the oven to 350°F (180°C/gas mark 4).

2. Oil a standard 9-inch loaf pan.

3. In a large bowl, mix the lemon zest and sugar.

4. Mix in the coconut oil. Stir the applesauce and lemon juice into the sugar mixture. Set aside.

5. In a medium bowl, whisk together the flour, baking powder, baking soda, and salt.

6. Mix the flour mixture into the sugar mixture.

7. Pour the batter into the oiled loaf pan.

8. Bake for 45 minutes, or until a toothpick inserted into the center of the cake comes out clean.

9. Cool the cake in the pan for 10 minutes, then remove it from the pan and let it cool completely on a cooling rack.

MAKE THE GLAZE (OPTIONAL)

10. In a small bowl, combine the sugar and lemon juice, and spoon over the cooled cake.

11. Spoon the glaze over the cooled cake.

PINEAPPLE UPSIDE-DOWN CAKE

MAKES 8 SERVINGS

I used to work in a senior center. One of our classes was woodworking. Everyone in the class was male, except for one woman, Helen. Helen loved to bake and brought delicious desserts with her every week. She was as sweet as her cakes, and she introduced me to desserts that would become some of my favorites, including Pineapple Upside-Down Cake. I updated Helen's recipe to incorporate slightly sweet, wholesome oat flour and coconut oil, rich in metabolism-boosting medium-chain fatty acids. I think Helen would be pleased with the results!

2½ teaspoons coconut oil, gently melted, divided

2   tablespoons brown sugar or coconut palm sugar

2   cups thinly sliced fresh pineapple

1½ cups (150 g) oat flour

⅓ cup (50g) evaporated cane juice or coconut palm sugar

1¾ teaspoons baking powder

¼ teaspoon salt

½ cup (125 g) applesauce

½ cup (120 mL) coconut milk

1   teaspoon vanilla extract

1   tablespoon apple cider vinegar

1. Preheat the oven to 375°F (190°C/gas mark 5).

2. Cover the bottom of a springform pan with a piece of parchment paper. Snap the sides onto the pan.

3. Spread ½ teaspoon melted coconut oil over the bottom of the parchment-lined pan and up the sides of the pan.

4. Sprinkle the brown sugar (or coconut palm sugar) over the bottom of the pan. Lay the pineapple slices in a single layer on top of the brown sugar.

5. In a medium bowl, whisk together the oat flour, evaporated cane juice (or coconut palm sugar), baking powder, and salt.

6. Mix in the applesauce, coconut milk, the remaining 2 teaspoons coconut oil, and the vanilla.

7. Stir the apple cider vinegar into the batter.

8. Pour the batter in the pan over the pineapple slices.

9. Bake for 30 minutes, or until a toothpick inserted into the center of the cake comes out clean.

10. Remove the cake and set it on a cooling rack. Loosen the sides of the springform pan. Let the cake cool 10 minutes.

11. Remove the sides of the pan. Invert the cake onto a serving plate.

OATMEAL CHOCOLATE CHIP ALMOND BUTTER COOKIES (CAN BE NUT-FREE)

MAKES 30 COOKIES

These cookies are wholesome enough for a special breakfast. They are rich in whole grains, and the nut butter (or sunflower seed butter) provides the fat instead of adding oil or butter. And, because they are sweetened with maple syrup, the cookies retain their rich, sweet moisture. To make them a great, nut-free snack to send along to school, too, just swap the almond butter with sunflower seed butter. Delicious. Note that the sunflower seed butter can react with the baking soda to give the cookies a greenish cast.

1 cup (100 g) oat flour (gluten-free, if necessary)

2 cups (160 g) rolled oats (gluten-free, if necessary)

½ teaspoon ground cinnamon

½ teaspoon baking soda

¼ teaspoon baking powder

½ teaspoon salt

½ cup (160 mL) maple syrup

½ cup (120 g) almond butter (or sunflower seed butter, if you need a nut-free option)

¾ cup (130 g) chocolate chips or chunks

1. Preheat the oven to 375°F (190°C/ gas mark 5). Line two baking sheets with parchment paper.

2. In a large bowl, whisk together the flour, oats, cinnamon, baking soda, baking powder, and salt.

3. In a medium bowl, add the almond butter to the maple syrup and stir to thoroughly combine.

4. Add the maple syrup mixture to the flour mixture and stir to combine.

5. Mix the chocolate chips into the batter.

6. Drop the batter by heaping tablespoonfuls onto the parchment-lined baking sheets.

7. Bake for 10 to 12 minutes, or until the cookies are set and golden.

8. Let the cookies cool on the baking sheet, set on cooling rack, for 5 minutes.

9. Remove the cookies from the sheet and set on the rack to cool completely.

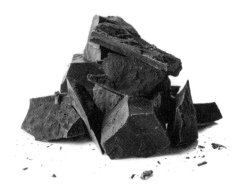

COCONUT MILLET PUDDING

MAKES 4 SERVINGS

This rice pudding uses whole-grain millet instead of refined white rice. The millet cooks up small and fluffy and makes for a pudding with a smooth texture. Coconut milk and vanilla (one of my favorite combinations) make the flavor of the pudding all the more delectable. If you want to jazz it up, mix in some fresh or frozen fruit—pineapples or cherries are nice options—or some nuts for crunch.

1 vanilla bean

3 cups (750 mL) canned coconut milk

⅔ cup (100 g) evaporated cane juice or coconut palm sugar

2 cups (350 g) prepared millet (page 24)

1. Slice the vanilla bean in half lengthwise. Using a small knife or spoon, scrape the seeds from the center of the vanilla bean and place in a medium-size saucepan.

2. Add the coconut milk and sugar. Mix until the sugar is dissolved.

3. Mix the millet into the coconut milk mixture.

4. Bring the mixture to a boil, reduce the heat, and simmer for 30 minutes.

5. Serve warm or cold.

WHOLE-GRAIN CHOCOLATE BROWNIES

MAKES 9 BROWNIES

These brownies get their chocolaty flavor from chocolate chips, so you know they are bursting with chocolate. The nut butter adds a complementary flavor that makes these brownies really special, and the protein and fiber from the whole grain–nut butter combination will keep you satisfied with one brownie, instead of feeling tempted to eat the whole pan. Chocolate-flavored nondairy yogurt (I like So Delicious chocolate-cultured coconut milk) will give these brownies an extra level of chocolate flavor.

- ¾ cup (100 g) evaporated cane juice or coconut palm sugar
- ½ cup (120 g) nut or seed butter (such as almond, peanut, or sunflower seed)
- 2 tablespoons water
- 2 cups (350 g) chocolate chips, divided
- 1½ teaspoons vanilla extract
- 1¼ cups (150 g) whole-grain spelt flour or (125 g) oat flour
- ½ teaspoon baking soda
- ½ teaspoon salt
- 1 6-ounce (170-g) container vanilla or chocolate nondairy yogurt

1. Preheat the oven to 350°F (180°C/gas mark 4). Line an 8- or 9-inch-square (20- or 23-cm) pan with parchment paper.

2. In a medium saucepan, combine the sugar, nut butter, and water.

3. Melt the mixture over medium heat until it is thoroughly combined.

4. Remove the saucepan from the heat and stir in half the chocolate chips until completely melted. Stir in the vanilla.

5. In a medium bowl, whisk together the flour, baking soda, and salt.

6. Mix the yogurt into the chocolate mixture.

7. Mix the chocolate mixture into the flour mixture. Stir the remaining chocolate chips into the batter.

8. Pour the batter into the parchment-lined pan.

9. Bake for 25 minutes, or until the brownies are set.

10. Let the brownies cool in the pan before cutting.

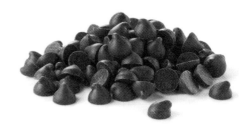

PEAR CRISP

MAKES 4 LARGE OR 6 MEDIUM SERVINGS

Why should apples get all of the crisp love? Pears are a wonderful fruit to bake with, too. In this recipe, the release of their sugary-sweet juices, combined with maple syrup, vanilla, and allspice, results in fruit nirvana. The addition of a crispy topping of oats and almonds elevates the dish to an even higher level of sumptuousness. If you want a creamy, cold contrast to the warm pears in this crisp, you can add a dollop of Maple Vanilla Ice Cream (page 98).

4 ripe pears (like Bartlett), thinly sliced

½ cup (75 g) evaporated cane juice or coconut palm sugar

1 teaspoon vanilla extract

2 tablespoons maple syrup

2 tablespoons neutral oil (sunflower, grapeseed, or canola)

½ cup (50 g) oat flour (gluten-free, if necessary)

¼ cup (20 g) rolled oats (gluten-free, if necessary)

¼ teaspoon ground allspice

¼ cup (25 g) slivered raw almonds

1. Preheat the oven to 400°F (200°C/gas mark 6).

2. Place the pear slices in a deep-dish pie plate or 9-inch cake pan.

3. In a large bowl, combine the sugar, vanilla, syrup, oil, flour, oats, allspice, and almonds.

4. Sprinkle the mixture on top of the pears.

5. Bake for 35 to 40 minutes, until the topping is set and golden, but not dark brown.

GLUTEN-FREE OATS

Oats are naturally gluten-free. Studies have shown, however, that commercially available oats are almost always contaminated with some gluten-containing grain. This contamination can happen at any time, starting from the field, where other cereal grains like wheat or barley might be intermingled with the oats, to the packaging, where dust containing gluten can be on the packaging equipment and may get mixed in with the oats. Because oats are such a nutrition powerhouse, several oat producers have taken steps to ensure that their oats remain gluten-free from field to package. If you need to avoid gluten, look for certified gluten-free oats to be sure that they are safe for you.

CHOCOLATE DONUTS

MAKES 6 DONUTS OR MUFFINS

One of my favorite kitchen purchases is a donut pan. If you don't have one of these specialized pans, you can still enjoy my recipe for Chocolate Donuts, which you can make in a muffin tin instead. Of course, this makes them muffins—not donuts—but they're just as delicious.

¼ cup (60 mL) olive oil, plus more
    for oiling

¾ cup (75 g) oat flour*

¼ cup (30 g) sweet white sorghum flour*

½ cup (75 g) evaporated cane juice or
    coconut palm sugar

¼ cup (20 g) cocoa powder

1¾ teaspoons baking powder

¼ teaspoon salt

¼ cup (65 g) applesauce

½ cup (120 mL) nondairy milk

½ teaspoon vanilla extract

½ teaspoon apple cider vinegar

¼ cup (50 g) chocolate chips

Note: If you don't need to use gluten-free flour, you can substitute 1 cup (120 g) whole-grain spelt flour for the ¾ cup oat flour and ¼ cup sorghum flour.

1. Preheat the oven to 350°F (180°C/gas mark 4). Lightly oil a donut (or muffin) pan.

2. In a medium bowl, whisk together the flours, sugar, cocoa, baking powder, and salt.

3. In a smaller bowl, combine the applesauce, nondairy milk, vanilla, apple cider vinegar, and ¼ cup olive oil.

4. Pour the applesauce mixture into the flour mixture and stir to combine.

5. Mix the chocolate chips into the batter.

6. Scoop the batter into a large resealable plastic bag or a pastry bag. If you're using a plastic bag, seal it, and snip off a bottom corner of the bag.

7. Pipe the batter into the donut or muffin pan, filling each cavity ⅔ full.

8. Bake the donuts for 12 to 14 minutes. A toothpick inserted into the middle of a donut should come out clean.

9. Let the donuts cool in the pan for a few minutes before transferring them to a cooling rack to cool completely.

SORGHUM FUN!

For over forty years, the town of Blairsville, Georgia, has hosted the Blairsville Sorghum Festival. Attendees can enjoy music, square dancing, biscuit eating, and all things sorghum. There is also a pageant that crowns a Miss Sorghum Festival.

PUMPKIN DONUTS

MAKES 6 DONUTS OR MUFFINS

Pumpkin isn't just the unofficial flavor of fall, it's also really good for you. Pumpkin, like other winter squashes, is an excellent source of vitamin A, vitamin C, and vitamin B6. Pumpkin donuts are a fun way to celebrate the flavor of the season when the weather starts to get cooler. If you need gluten-free donuts, simply substitute oat flour and sorghum flour for the spelt flour, as noted below.

¼ cup (60 mL) olive oil, plus more for oiling

1 cup (120 g) whole-grain spelt flour*

1¾ teaspoons baking powder, divided

¼ teaspoon salt

¼ teaspoon ground nutmeg

½ teaspoon ground cinnamon

½ cup (125 g) canned pumpkin (or cooked and pureed)

½ cup (75 g) evaporated cane juice or coconut palm sugar

½ cup (120 mL) nondairy milk (unflavored or vanilla)

½ teaspoon vanilla extract

½ teaspoon apple cider vinegar

*Note: For gluten-free donuts, substitute ¾ cup (25 g) gluten-free oat flour and ¼ cup (30 g) sweet white sorghum flour for the spelt flour.

1. Preheat the oven to 350°F (180°C/gas mark 4). Lightly oil a donut pan or muffin tin.

2. In a medium bowl, whisk together the flour, 1¼ teaspoons baking powder, salt, nutmeg, and cinnamon.

3. In a large bowl, combine the pumpkin with the remaining ½ teaspoon of baking powder.

4. Mix the sugar, nondairy milk, vanilla, apple cider vinegar, and ¼ cup olive oil into the pumpkin mixture.

5. Add the flour mixture to the pumpkin mixture and stir well to combine.

6. Scoop the batter into a large resealable plastic bag or a pastry bag. If you're using a plastic bag, seal it and snip off a bottom corner of the bag.

7. Pipe the batter into the donut or muffin pan, filling each cavity ⅔ full.

7. Bake for 10 minutes. The batter should be set and the top should be dry, but the donuts will be fragile.

8. Let the donuts cool in the pan for 5 minutes before gently removing them to a cooling rack to cool completely.

STRAWBERRY OATMEAL ICE CREAM

MAKES 6 TO 8 SERVINGS

I love oat milk, so I knew I'd love oatmeal ice cream. My friend Kristina Sloggett, from the gorgeous website SpaBettie, makes a decadent chocolate ice cream from oats, so I knew it could be done—and taste delicious. You can make this ice cream in an ice cream maker or you can freeze it in ice pop molds. It definitely has an oat flavor, which I enjoy, but you can reduce the oats to a half cup if you'd like the flavor less pronounced.

1   cup (80 g) rolled oats

3   cups (450 g) strawberries (fresh or frozen)

1   15-ounce can (about 400 mL) full-fat coconut milk

¼   cup (50 mL) agave nectar

1. In a medium bowl, cover the oats with fresh water and set aside to soak, covered loosely with a plate or kitchen towel, for at least 4 hours. Drain the oats.

2. In a blender, place the oats, strawberries, coconut milk, and agave nectar. Blend until the oats are completely broken down.

3. If using an ice cream maker, chill the mixture in the refrigerator for at least 1 hour, then follow the manufacturer's instructions for using the ice cream maker.

4. If using ice pop molds to make ice cream bars, pour the mixture into molds and freeze until solid.

MAPLE VANILLA ICE CREAM

MAKES 4 SERVINGS OR 8 BARS

If you use an ice cream maker to make this recipe, you can serve it with Pear Crisp (page 95) or Maple Bourbon Bread Pudding (page 102) for a really decadent dessert. If you don't have an ice cream maker, this recipe can be used to make wonderfully creamy ice cream bars—just make sure your molds are stainless steel or BPA-free plastic (you don't want dangerous chemicals to leach into your food!).

1   cup (80 g) rolled oats

1   cup (250 mL) water

1   teaspoon vanilla extract

½   teaspoon ground cinnamon

3   tablespoons maple syrup

1   6-ounce container (170 g) vanilla nondairy yogurt (coconut milk yogurt is also really nice)

1. In a medium bowl, cover the oats with fresh water and set aside to soak, covered loosely with a plate or kitchen towel, for at

ICE CREAM EQUIPMENT

INSTANT ICE CREAM

If you don't have an ice cream maker, you can use ice pop molds to create "ice cream" bars. Your icy treat will freeze a little harder in an ice pop mold than it would in an ice cream maker, because you don't get the same introduction of air that makes for a fluffy ice cream, but it will taste just as good. If you don't have an ice pop mold, you can make your own with a paper cup. Pour the mixture into the cup, cover it with foil, and insert a popsicle stick through the foil into the center of the mixture. When the mixture is frozen, remove the foil and peel away the cup, revealing your homemade ice pop. Enjoy!

HOW TO CHOOSE AN ICE POP MOLD

You can buy ice pop molds (or popsicle molds) almost anywhere kitchen tools are sold—at a big box store or at your local grocery store. You can also buy specialty ice pop makers online or at fancy kitchen stores. The wide range of prices for molds can make it difficult to decide which to buy: should you spend more on an ice pop system or go for the cheapest option at the dollar store? There are a couple of important things to consider before you make a choice. Ice pop molds are made from either plastic or stainless steel. If you're buying plastic molds, look for ones that say "BPA Free." BPA (or bisphenol A), a toxic compound found in many plastics, can leach into food, especially if the mold has been heated—in the dishwasher, for example. To avoid this, look for BPA-free or stainless steel ice pop molds.

I like ice pop setups that allow you to fill individual molds. Mine has a stand with four separate molds. I can make just one ice pop or four, depending on how much liquid I have. This is especially handy for freezing a little leftover smoothie into an ice pop. I can get fruits and even veggies into my kids with a smoothie ice pop, and they just think they're having a treat!

least 4 hours. Most of the liquid should be absorbed, but drain off any excess liquid.

2. Blend all the ingredients (including 1 cup fresh water) together in a blender until smooth.

3. If using an ice cream maker, chill the mixture in the refrigerator for 1 hour, then follow the manufacturer's instructions for using the ice cream maker.

4. If using ice pop molds to make ice cream bars, pour the mixture into molds and freeze until solid.

COCONUT-OIL SPELT PIECRUST

MAKES 2 CRUSTS

Lots of people are intimidated by the idea of making their own piecrust. It doesn't need to be so! This ancient grain crust is easy to make and very forgiving. The whole-grain spelt in this recipe has a nutty flavor, but isn't as heavy as whole wheat.

2½ cups (300 g) whole-grain spelt flour

1 tablespoon evaporated cane juice or coconut palm sugar

1 teaspoon salt

1 cup (220 g) coconut oil, soft, but firm

½ cup (125 mL) ice water

1. In a large shallow bowl, whisk together the flour, sugar, and salt.

2. Cut the coconut oil into the flour mixture with a pastry cutter or two knives. There should still be some visible (pea-size) chunks of flour-coated oil in the mix.

3. Add the ice water, but not the ice, to the mixture one tablespoon at a time. Use a rubber spatula or wooden spoon to thoroughly combine the mixture.

4. Once the dough holds together, form it into two disks.*

5. Roll out the dough, one disk at a time, on a floured board or counter.

6. Transfer each disk to a pie pan or follow directions below for freezing crust for later use.

7. Bake piecrust according to your pie recipe.

*If you're not going to use the dough right away, wrap it tightly in plastic wrap and store it in the freezer for up to 3 months. Thaw the dough before rolling it out.

COCONUT OIL WITHOUT THE COCONUT FLAVOR

Everyone has a food that he or she really can't stand. For my sister, it's coconut. If I try to sneak a little coconut into a cookie, my sister can taste it, even if no one else can. That led me to ask the question: Is it possible to get the healthy fats and lovely texture of coconut oil without the coconut flavor? Fortunately for my sister, the answer is yes. While unrefined coconut oil has a light coconut flavor, refined coconut oil has the healthy medium-chain fatty acids of its unrefined relative, without any coconut flavor or aroma. Coconut oil is an ideal fat for baking because it gives cakes, pies, and biscuits a tender crumb with a melt-in-your-mouth texture.

BLUEBERRY PIE WITH WHOLE-GRAIN CRUST

MAKES 8 SERVINGS

In this recipe, the whole-grain spelt crust counterbalances the sweet, juicy blueberries, resulting in a really balanced pie. If your berries are tart, add a little more sugar. The starch helps thicken the juices so that the pie will slice nicely.

- 4   *cups (600 g) fresh blueberries*
- 2   *tablespoons evaporated cane juice or coconut palm sugar*
- 2   *teaspoons fresh lemon juice*
- 2   *tablespoons potato starch or cornstarch*
- 2   *whole-grain Coconut-oil Spelt Piecrusts (page 100)*

1. Preheat the oven to 375°F (190°C/gas mark 5).

2. In a large bowl, combine the blueberries, sugar, lemon juice, and starch. Mix together.

3. Roll out one crust and place it in the bottom of a standard 9-inch (23-cm) pie plate.

4. Pour the blueberry mixture on top of the crust.

5. Roll out the second crust and place it on top of the pie. Crimp the edges together. Cut 4 to 6 slits into the top of the piecrust.

6. Bake for 45 to 50 minutes, or until the pie is golden and juices are bubbling through the slits.

7. Allow the pie to cool before slicing.

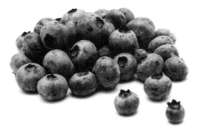

MAPLE BOURBON BREAD PUDDING

MAKES 8 SERVINGS

Chicago-based Koval Distillery makes excellent bourbon using one of my favorite ancient grains—millet—which inspired me to incorporate bourbon in a recipe for bread pudding that's the perfect ending to a hearty, cold-weather dinner. Even better, serve some warm Maple Bourbon Bread Pudding in a bowl topped with Maple Oat Ice Cream (page 98).

1   cup (160 g) cashews
1   cup (250 mL) boiling water
1   cup (300 mL) maple syrup
¼   cup (60 mL) bourbon (preferably Koval)
¼   cup (35 g) brown sugar
1   tablespoon vanilla extract
½   loaf Spelt Oat Bread (page 72) or
     Spelt Sandwich Loaf (page 73), torn
     into approximately 1½-inch pieces
     (approximately 6 cups, or about 300 g)

1. Preheat the oven to 375°F (190°C/gas mark 5).

2. Place the cashews in a large bowl.

3. Pour the boiling water over the cashews. Cover the bowl with a plate or kitchen towel, and set aside for 10 minutes.

4. Using a blender, blend together the cashews, soaking water, maple syrup, bourbon, brown sugar, and vanilla.

5. Spread the bread pieces over the bottom of a casserole dish or 9 × 13-inch (22 × 33-cm) baking pan.

6. Pour the cashew mixture over the bread. Make sure that all the bread is coated with liquid.

7. Bake, uncovered, for 45 minutes. The bread pudding should be golden brown with slightly crispy edges.

A TOAST TO ANCIENT GRAINS

Bourbon is a whiskey distilled from corn. Most bourbons also include wheat or rye as a supplement. However, at Chicago craft distillery Koval, which turns organic grains into high-end spirits, millet supplements the corn instead of wheat or rye. Koval also makes whiskey from another favorite ancient grain, oats. Corsair Distillery in Tennessee is also experimenting with the flavors that ancient grains offer, creating high-end spirits using oats, spelt, and others. High West, a distillery in Park City, Utah, is also transforming oats into high-end liquor. The next time you have a celebratory sip, try millet bourbon or oat whiskey. I think you'll like it. Bottoms up!

MUG BROWNIE

MAKES 1 BROWNIE

I love chocolate, and sometimes nothing else will satisfy my sweet tooth. This mini mug brownie allows me to indulge in a chocolate cake, but not overindulge. Making just a single serving means that I won't have to resist leftovers later.

4   *tablespoons evaporated cane juice or coconut palm sugar*

4   *tablespoons oat flour*

2   *tablespoons cocoa powder*

1   *tablespoon coconut oil*

1   *tablespoon applesauce*

2   *tablespoons water*

Pinch of salt

1. Combine all the ingredients in a microwave-safe bowl or mug (or an oven-safe bowl or mug if you are using an oven).

2. Stir to thoroughly mix all the ingredients.

3. Microwave the brownie mixture on high for 1 minute; or, if you're using an oven, bake the mixture in a 350°F (175°C/gas mark 4) preheated oven for 10 to 15 minutes, or until a toothpick inserted into the center of the brownie comes out clean.

4. Let the brownie cool a little before eating it, as it will be quite hot.

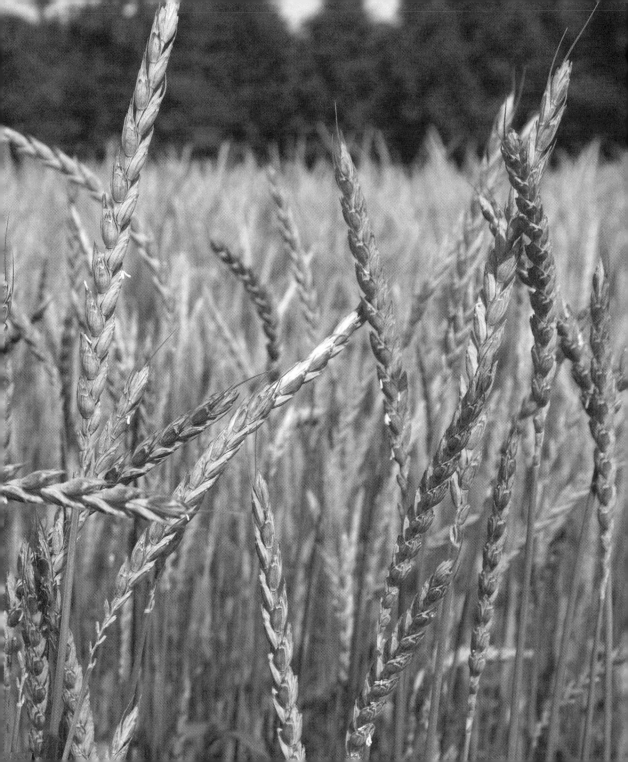

CHAPTER 9

FREQUENTLY ASKED QUESTIONS

Between my blog and the presentations I give, I receive many questions about the ingredients I use. Some questions about ancient grains come up again and again. Whether folks want to know about the health benefits of these grains or how to begin using or storing them, these are some of the questions that I am most frequently asked.

What are the main nutrients in millet?

Millet is a good source of protein, fiber, magnesium, phosphorus, copper, thiamine (vitamin B1), and niacin (vitamin B3). It is also an excellent source of manganese.

What are the main nutrients in oats?

Oats are a good source of protein, fiber, iron, magnesium, phosphorus, zinc, copper, selenium, and thiamine (vitamin B1), as well as an excellent source of manganese.

What are the main nutrients in spelt and farro?

Spelt and farro are good sources of protein, fiber, iron, magnesium, phosphorus, zinc, copper, thiamine (vitamin B1), niacin (vitamin B3), and manganese.

What are the main nutrients in sorghum?

Sorghum is a good source of fiber, magnesium, phosphorus, selenium, and

niacin (vitamin B3), and an excellent source of manganese.

What are the main nutrients in teff?

Teff has more calcium than any other grain. One cup of cooked teff has about the same amount of calcium as ½ cup of cooked spinach. Teff is also a good source of protein, fiber, iron, magnesium, phosphorus, zinc, thiamine (vitamin B1), and pyridoxine (vitamin B6). It is also an excellent source of copper and manganese.

What are the health benefits of the vitamins and minerals found in ancient grains?

PROTEIN: Protein is essential for cell development and repair, as well as for growth and development at all stages of life.

FIBER: Dietary fiber is very important for digestive health and regular bowel movements. It also helps your body slow down the digestion of starches and sugars, and this can lower cholesterol in your blood over time, thereby reducing your risk of heart disease and stroke. It can also help with glucose tolerance in people with diabetes.

MANGANESE: Manganese plays a role in forming healthy bones, connective tissue, and sex hormones. Low levels of manganese can be a contributing factor to infertility.

MAGNESIUM: Every organ in your body, including your heart, liver, and lungs, needs magnesium, which also helps balance levels of other important nutrients in your body. Magnesium intake has been shown, in some studies, to improve conditions as varied as restless legs syndrome, high blood pressure, and noise-related hearing loss.

PHOSPHORUS: Phosphorus is an important component of teeth and bones. It can also help lessen muscle discomfort after a hard workout.

COPPER: Copper plays a crucial role in creating red blood cells and keeping your immune and nervous systems healthy. It is also a key component of collagen, an essential part of your bones and connective tissue.

IRON: Iron is critical for healthy red blood cells, which carry oxygen-rich blood to every part of your body. Anemia can result from inadequate iron in the blood and can lead to fatigue and lethargy.

ZINC: Zinc is present in every cell of your body. It helps keep your immune system healthy and plays an important part in keeping your senses working well, as it is key to smell, taste, and vision.

SELENIUM: Selenium promotes a healthy immune system and a smoothly functioning thyroid. It is also an antioxidant that can help counteract damage caused by pollution and aging.

THIAMINE (VITAMIN B1): Thiamine helps your body transform carbohydrates into energy.

NIACIN (VITAMIN B3): Niacin helps your skin, digestive system, and nervous system to function well. It also plays a role in converting the food you eat into energy.

PYRIDOXINE (VITAMIN B6): Pyridoxine is important for brain development and function and plays a role in regulating mood and your body clock.

What is the best way to store my grains?

Because grains can go rancid more quickly than you might think, it is a good idea to store them in an airtight container in the refrigerator or freezer. This will keep them fresher longer. I keep my grains in the freezer for up to three months. Oats are the exception to this rule; because they have been lightly roasted before you purchase them, they will stay fresher longer. Oats can stay fresh for up to one year (though mine never last that long!).

Is there a difference between rolled oats and old-fashioned oats?

Rolled oats and old-fashioned oats are two different names for the same thing.

Which ancient grains are gluten-free?

Millet, sorghum, teff, and oats are naturally gluten-free. If you need your grain to be gluten-free, look for a certified gluten-free label to be sure that it is safe for you, because grains can be contaminated with gluten by coming in contact with other grains at any stage in the process of traveling from field to mill.

Why is spelt labeled as containing wheat on food allergy labels?

In January 2006, the Food Allergy Labeling and Consumer Protection Act came into effect. This law requires that food manufacturers label common allergens (eggs, milk, tree nuts, peanuts, shellfish, fish, wheat, and soy) on ingredient lists in the United States. Spelt is required by this law to be labeled as wheat. Because spelt is related to wheat, some people who are allergic to wheat might be allergic to spelt, too. If you are allergic to wheat, it is best to consult your doctor before you eat spelt.

Are spelt and farro the same thing?

No. Both spelt and farro are descendants of einkorn, as is modern wheat. They have different DNA structures. Farro has fewer chromosomes than spelt. Although they are different, sometimes they are sold with farro labeled as spelt, or vice versa.

How can I substitute gluten-free oat flour for all-purpose wheat flour?

You can substitute gluten-free oat flour for all-purpose wheat flour one for one in your baking. Because oats have a similar protein structure to the gluten in wheat, you will not need a binder like xanthan gum or guar gum to hold your baked goods together. It's important to remember, though, that there will be some differences when you switch to a whole-grain flour like oat flour from a processed flour like all-purpose wheat flour. First, there will be some changes in texture. Oat flour has a higher moisture content than wheat flour. Also, the protein bonds are not quite as strong in oat flour as in wheat flour, so your baked goods will be slightly more tender when you make the change. Second, your baked goods will be more nutritious. All of the fiber is ground into oat flour, but all-purpose wheat flour has the fiber stripped away before it's ground. Finally, your baked goods will have a lovely oat-tinged flavor that makes muffins, cookies, and cakes even more delicious.

Why can some people tolerate the gluten in spelt and farro, even though they are intolerant of the gluten in wheat?

Spelt, farro, and wheat all come from the same ancestor grain, einkorn. Farro, or emmer as it's also known, is an early variant of einkorn; spelt is a later variety; and modern wheat is the result of both natural and artificial hybridization. Over time, genetic modifications have resulted in related but different plants. Modern wheat has been manipulated to produce the highest yields and to be the easiest to harvest of all the grain cousins. Along with changes in how the plant looks and how the grain is collected, however, structural changes to the proteins and other components of the grain have occurred. Therefore, although spelt, farro, and modern wheat all contain gluten, the gluten molecules are not the same from grain variety to grain variety. These changes mean that some people who have trouble digesting modern wheat do not have the same digestive discomfort when they eat spelt or farro. For people with a wheat allergy or celiac disease (an autoimmune disorder that requires avoiding gluten), spelt and farro should also be avoided unless a doctor advises otherwise.

Do I need to presoak grains before cooking them?

Millet, teff, sorghum, farro, and oats can be cooked right away. Spelt has a tougher exterior that requires soaking for between 4 to 8 hours (or even overnight) before cooking, unless you are using a slow cooker. If you are using a slow cooker to prepare spelt, you do not need to presoak it.

Are ancient grains good sources of fiber?

If you are enjoying ancient grains as whole grains, they are all great sources of fiber. Spelt flour is available in white and whole-grain versions, so if you want the fiber benefits of a whole-grain flour, you need to check the label on the package. It should say "whole spelt" or "whole-grain spelt" in the ingredient list, if it's a whole grain.

Can I substitute sorghum flour for all-purpose wheat flour?

No. Sorghum flour can be a flavorful and nutritious addition to a gluten-free flour blend, but it should make up only approximately 20 percent of the overall flour mix. You need to blend it with other lighter flours and/or starches to get baked goods with a consistency that is appealing. When used as part of a gluten-free blend, though, the higher protein content of sorghum flour, along with its pleasantly nutty flavor, will enhance your baking. I like to mix some sorghum flour into my oat flour for a versatile gluten-free flour blend that doesn't need an additional binder.

What are the benefits of adding oats to my smoothies?

I love smoothies as a complete meal in a glass. I can mix up a combination of fruits, vegetables, seeds, and nuts and provide my family with a great start to the day or a re-energizing after-school snack. Adding rolled oats into the mixture ensures that I will have the energy I need to accomplish my goals for hours. The fiber in oats keeps me from feeling hungry too soon, and the complex carbohydrates provide slow-burning energy that lasts for hours, without the sugar crash that can come from energy drinks.

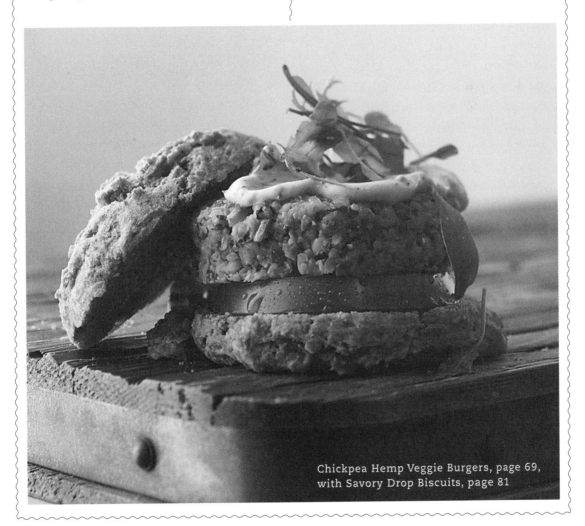

Chickpea Hemp Veggie Burgers, page 69, with Savory Drop Biscuits, page 81

What are the advantages of using prepared millet instead of uncooked millet when making foods with tomatoes?

You might have noticed that in all of the recipes in this book that feature millet and tomatoes, prepared millet is in the ingredient list. I learned the hard way that when you try to cook millet in water that includes tomatoes, the millet will not cook—it never softens and fluffs. Instead, the little balls of millet remain hard. It's easy to remedy this problem, though. When making a tomato and millet-based recipe, like Salsa Millet Hash (page 34) or Millet and Poblano Chili (page 46), you just need to cook the millet separately. Once it's cooked, the millet can be incorporated into the dish.

Is it better to use rolled oats or steel-cut oats?

The type of oat you choose depends on what you are using it for. Steel-cut oats work well in oatmeal made in a slow cooker, because they have a sturdier structure that can stand up to hours of low heat. If you use rolled oats in a slow cooker, they will break down and you will end up with mush, instead of a well-textured breakfast cereal. Rolled oats are a better choice when you're blending oats, because their thinner texture will break up more thoroughly. When you're making a creamy soup or blending oats into a smoothie, rolled oats are the preferred choice. Whichever you choose, rolled oats or steel-cut oats, you get similar health benefits.

Are amaranth and quinoa ancient grains?

Ancient grains, like all grains, are the seeds of cereal plants, which are a type of grass. Amaranth and quinoa are considered pseudo-grains, because, although they have strong nutrition profiles and can often be used in conjunction with or in place of grains, they are the seeds of other types of plants. For information on how to incorporate amaranth and quinoa into a healthy diet, please check my previous book, *Super Seeds* (Sterling 2014), which is filled with recipes, facts, and tips about quinoa and amaranth, as well as chia, flax, and hemp.

Is buckwheat a form of wheat?

Despite its name, buckwheat is a seed that is actually a relative of rhubarb and sorrel. It is not a cereal grain, like wheat or its ancient relatives, spelt and farro. Buckwheat is a gluten-free grain alternative that can play an important role in gluten-free baking and cooking.

While writing this book, I learned so much about how ancient grains can keep our bodies strong and healthy. These studies provided invaluable information about the role of ancient grains in our history and our health:

Satya S. Jonnalagadda, Lisa Harnack, Rui Hai Liu, Nicola McKeown, Chris Seal, Simin Liu, and George C. Fahey. "Putting the Whole Grain Puzzle Together: Health Benefits Associated with Whole Grain—Summary of American Society for Nutrition 2010 Satellite Symposium," *The Journal of Nutrition Supplement 141*, no. 2 (2011): 1011S-1022S.

Nicola M. McKeown, Lisa M. Troy, Paul F. Jacques, Udo Hoffmann, Christopher J. O'Donnell, and Caroline S. Fox. "Whole- and Refined-Grain Intakes Are Differentially Associated with Abdominal Visceral and Subcutaneous Adiposity in Healthy Adults: the Framingham Heart Study," *The American Journal of Clinical Nutrition* 92, no. 5 (2010): 1165-1171.

Mette Kristensen, Søren Toubro, Morten Georg Jensen, Alastair B. Ross, Giancarlo Riboldi, Michela Petronio, Susanne Bügel, Inge Tetens, and Arne Astrup. "Whole Grain Compared with Refined Wheat Decreases the Percentage of Body Fat Following a 12-Week, Energy-Restricted Dietary Intervention in Postmenopausal Women," *The Journal of Nutrition 142*, no. 4 (2012): 710-6.

The resources below provided me with a great deal of information, as well, and they can be a valuable resource for you, too.

www.umm.edu
The University of Maryland Medical Center's Medical Encyclopedia provides a lot of information about various nutrients and how they function to promote human health.

www.nutritiondata.self.com
SELF Nutrition Data allows you to type in a food or ingredient to find out its nutrient makeup and nutritional strengths.

www.whfoods.com
The World's Healthiest Foods ranks foods in terms of healthfulness, and it offers a lot of information, recipes, and other resources on how to eat healthfully.

ods.od.nih.gov
The Office of Dietary Supplements at the National Institutes of Health has nutrient research that is presented for laypeople.

www.wholegrainscouncil.org
The Whole Grains Council offers information—including nutrition, recipes, and other resources—about a variety of whole grains.

KITCHEN RESOURCES

Black and Decker
www.blackanddeckerappliances.com
Black and Decker makes a wide range of appliances, including slow cookers, waffle irons, blenders, griddles, and more.

Blendtec
www.blendtec.com
Blendtec produces high-speed, powerful blenders.

Calphalon
www.calphalon.com
Calphalon manufactures a complete range of outstanding bakeware, cookware, and cutlery.

Cuisinart
www.cuisinart.com
Cuisinart makes a full line of kitchen appliances, including blenders, food processors, immersion blenders, ice cream makers, and more.

Hamilton Beach
www.hamiltonbeach.com
Hamilton Beach produces a complete line of appliances, including blenders, ice cream makers, slow cookers, food processors, waffle irons, and more.

KitchenAid
www.kitchenaid.com

KitchenAid offers a complete line of kitchen appliances, including stand mixers, blenders, coffee grinders, waffle makers, food processors, and more.

Vitamix
www.vitamix.com

Vitamix produces high-speed, powerful blenders.

SUPPLIERS OF ANCIENT GRAINS

You can find ancient grains in most well-stocked grocery stores, health food stores, and online. Here are some of my favorite brands/suppliers.

Arrowhead Mills
www.arrowheadmills.com

Millet flour, spelt and oat flour, and millet grain.

Bob's Red Mill
www.bobsredmill.com

A full line of ancient grains and ancient-grain flours.

Gerbs
www.mygerbs.com

Gluten-free, allergen-free ancient grains: millet, sorghum, and teff.

Pacific Foods
www.pacificfoods.com

Packaged oat milk.

Windy City Cocoa
www.windycitycocoa.com

Dairy-free instant hot cocoa made with oats.

SPIRITS WITH ANCIENT GRAINS

Corsair Distillery
www.corsairdistillery.com

Spirits distilled using oats, spelt, and other ancient grains.

High West Distillery and Saloon
www.highwest.com

Spirits distilled with oats.

Koval
www.koval-distillery.com

Spirits distilled with millet and oats.

ABOUT THE AUTHOR

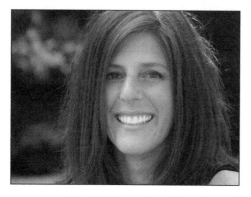

KIM LUTZ is a Chicago-based author and the founder of Kim's Welcoming Kitchen (welcomingkitchen.com) and the WINDY CITY COCOA brand of all-natural, dairy-free instant hot cocoa and dessert mix (www.windycitycocoa.com). She is a contributor to the influential Disney and Mylan website, My Allergy Kingdom. Lutz is the author of *Welcoming Kitchen: 200 Delicious Allergen and Gluten-free Vegan Recipes* (Sterling Publishing) and *Super Seeds* (Sterling Publishing) and co-author of *The Everything Organic Cooking for Baby and Toddler Book* and *The Everything Guide to Cooking for Children with Autism*. Lutz has been featured in the *Chicago Sun-Times*, *Chicago Parent*, on WGN-TV, and FOX Chicago, among other media.

ACKNOWLEDGMENTS

I am so grateful to the many people who helped make *Ancient Grains* a reality. My guys—Steve, Casey, and Evan—have been so patient with all of the recipe testing, tasting, hits and misses, messy kitchen, and so much more that came with this project. My family and friends are probably the most supportive people out there; without their support, I couldn't have done this. Julie Han kept me on track and organized. I'd still be recipe-testing without her!

This book is so much better thanks to the efforts of an amazing group of recipe testers. Thank you to Michelle Bishop, Heather Rossman, Tammy Azzarello, Michele Ritchie, Nancy Konstantos, Dana Murray, Robin Karlov, Valerie Hedge, Ana Breen, Jo-Ann LaPorta, Madeleine Pearl, Julie Brown, Kirsten Lambert, Kevin Sullivan, Angel Li, Laura Sagami, Ilene Mash, Stefanie Dopp, Lisa Miranda, Karen Plumley, Liz Uligian, and Julie Han.

I am also so grateful to the talented and supportive people at Sterling Publishing. Jennifer Williams is such a warm and wonderful editor. I am so glad we worked together again on this book. Hannah Reich made this book so much better with her thoughtful questions and edits. Thanks also to designers Christine Heun and Barbara Balch, and to Marilyn Kretzer, Sterling's editorial director.

INDEX

Note: Page numbers in *italics* indicate photos on pages separate from recipes.

Almonds. *See* Nuts and seeds
Amaranth, 3, 110
Ancient grains. *See also* specific grains
  amaranth and, 3, 110
  in Bible, 71
  biofuels from, 4, 5
  historical perspective, 1
  introduction to, 2–13
  in the morning, 31. *See also* Breakfast
  nutritional/health benefits, 17–19
  powering up workouts, 40
  quinoa and, 3, 110
  resources, 112–113
  seeds compared to, 3
  spirits with, 102, 113
  storing, 43, 106–107
  substitution flexibility, 22
  texture appeal, 22
  today, 1–2
  traveling with, 82
  whole grain benefits, 15–16
Apricot-Dijon Vinaigrette, 50
Artichokes
  Artichoke Farro (or Sorghum), *52*, 66
  Hummus Arugula Flatbread, 68
  Lemon Artichoke Hummus, 68
Asparagus Sorghum Sauté, 54

Baked goods, 71–83
  about: baking vs. nutritional yeast, 55; flatbread options/ suggestions, 79; overview of recipes, 71; slicing bread or not, 72; substituting gluten-free oat flour for wheat flour, 107
  Blueberry Scones, 75
  Chocolate Chip Scones, *70*, 74
  Flatbread Croutons, 48–49
  Garlic Flatbread, 78
  Gluten-free Beer Bread, 77
  Maple Bourbon Bread Pudding, 102
  Multigrain Gluten-free Biscuits, 78–79

Peach Mango Muffins, 82
  Savory Drop Biscuits, 81, *109*
  Spelt Oat Bread, 72
  Spelt Sandwich Loaf, 73
  Spelt Tortillas or Flatbreads, 76
  Tender Cornbread, 80
Banana, in Creamy Sunrise Smoothie, 36
Basic recipes, 21–27
  about: overview of, 21
  Basic Farro, 24
  Basic Millet, 24
  Basic Overnight Oats, 30
  Basic Teff, 25
  Oat Flour, 25
  Oat Milk, 27
  Prepared Sorghum, 22
  Slow Cooker Spelt, 23
  Sorghum Popcorn, 22
  Spelt, Stove-Top Method, 23
Batch cooking, 30
Beans and other legumes
  about: pulse nutritional/health benefits, 62
  Chickpea Hemp Veggie Burgers, 69, *109*
  Hummus Arugula Flatbread, 68
  Lemon Artichoke Hummus, 68
  Lemon Dill Grain Salad, *42*, 48
  Millet and Poblano Chili, 46–47
  Multigrain Veggie Burger Crumbles, 62
  Quick Farro Risotto, 56
  Teff-Lentil Sloppy Joes, 63
Beer bread, gluten-free, 77
Bell Pepper Cashew Sauce, 60
Berries
  about: blending with oat milk cubes, 27; nutritional benefits, 32; strawberries, 32
  Blueberry Pie with Whole-Grain Crust, 101
  Blueberry Scones, 75
  Creamy Sunrise Smoothie, 36
  Raspberry Chocolate Chip Cake, 86–87
  Strawberry Oatmeal Ice Cream, 98

Strawberry Waffles, 32
  Where's the Green? Smoothie, 35
Birds, whole grains for, 45
Biscuits. *See* Baked goods
Blenders, 37
Blueberries. *See* Berries
Bourbon, in Maple Bourbon Bread Pudding, 102
Bourbons, from ancient grains, 102
BPA (bisphenol-A) alternatives, 61
Breads. *See* Baked goods
Breakfast, 29–41
  about: adding oats to smoothies, 109; ancient grains for, 31; kid-friendly recipes, 36; overview of recipes, 29
  Basic Overnight Oats, 30
  Cinnamon Mug Coffee Cake, 41
  Cocoa Power Bites, 40
  Creamy Sunrise Smoothie, 36
  Egg-free French Toast, 38
  Millet Porridge, 30
  Nutty Granola, *28*, 39
  Pancakes, 31
  Peach Almond Overnight Oatmeal, 39
  Portable Oatmeal, 33
  Salsa Millet Hash, 34
  Slow Cooker Steel-cut Maple and Brown Sugar Oats, 34
  Strawberry Waffles, 32
  Where's the Green? Smoothie, 35
Brussels Sprouts Millet Slaw, 49
Buckwheat, 110

Cakes. *See* Desserts
Cancer, grains and, ix, xi, 15, 18
Cashews. *See* Nuts and seeds
Cats, oat grass for, 35
Chickpeas. *See* Beans and other legumes
Chili, millet and poblano, 46–47
Chocolate
  about: health benefits of, 86; Windy City Cocoa, 41
  Chocolate Chip Scones, *70*, 74
  Chocolate Donuts, *84*, 96

(continued)

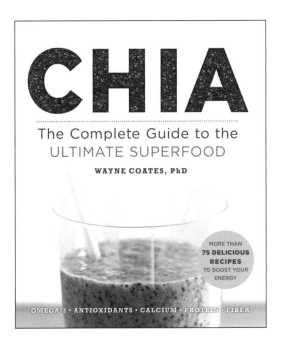

CHIA

The Complete Guide to the Ultimate Superfood
Wayne Coates, PhD, with Stephanie Pedersen
978-1-4027-9943-3

Chia is the little miracle seed for anyone trying to lose weight, stay healthy, and enhance well-being. Used by the Aztecs for centuries, it's a gluten-free natural appetite suppressant that helps regenerate muscle, sustain energy, and balance blood sugar. This definitive work explains all you need to know about chia, and provides a comprehensive daily strategy for weight loss with delicious recipes!

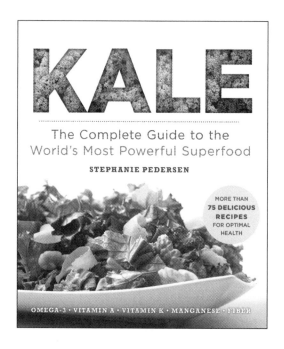

KALE

The Complete Guide to the World's Most Powerful Superfood
Stephanie Pedersen
978-1-4549-0625-4

From farmers and foodies to celebrity chefs—everyone's gone mad for kale! For those eager to get in on this healthy, tasty trend, here is a fun-to-read, one-stop resource for all things kale, including more than 75 delicious recipes to entice, satisfy, and boost well-being. Stephanie Pedersen, a holistic health counselor, provides dozens of tips for making kale delicious and desirable to even the most finicky eater.

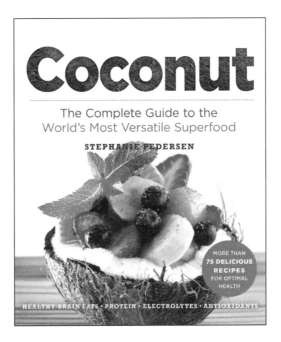

COCONUT

The Complete Guide to the World's Most Versatile Superfood
Stephanie Pedersen
978-1-4549-1340-5

Perfect for dishes both savory and sweet, coconut is delicious—and, even better, it's a nutritional powerhouse with myriad health benefits. Find out how to choose, use, and store every bit of the coconut, along with more than 75 recipes that make you feel as good as they taste. And, in addition to informative sidebars, there's advice on making coconut-based beauty supplies!

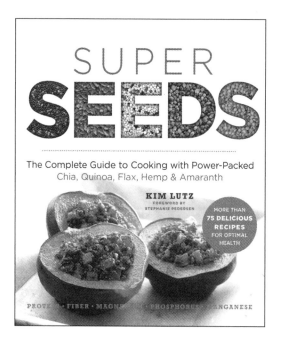

SUPER SEEDS

The Complete Guide to Cooking with Power-Packed Chia,
Quinoa, Flax, Hemp & Amaranth

Kim Lutz

978-1-4549-1278-1

Five super seeds—in one super volume! Chia, hemp, flax, quinoa, and amaranth are tiny powerhouses that deliver whopping amounts of protein, essential fatty acids, and great taste in every serving. Perfect for vegan and gluten-free diets, they're the stars of these 75 mouthwatering recipes. Essential for anyone interested in eating healthily . . . and deliciously.

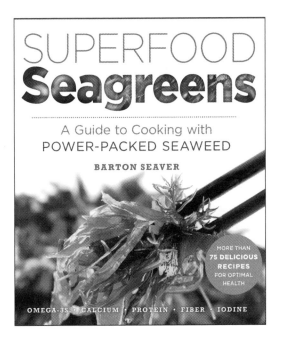

SUPERFOOD SEAGREENS

The Guide to Cooking with Power-Packed Seaweed
Barton Seaver
978-1-4549-1739-7

It's no wonder that seagreens (such as dulse, kelp, and wakame) are poised to become the next superfood craze, given their amazing health benefits. Now you can incorporate them into your daily diet—with the help of world-renowned chef and sustainability expert Barton Seaver. More than 75 versatile recipes include everything from smoothies and cocktails to exciting salads, delicious pasta dishes, savory stews and soups, and even breakfast foods and desserts.

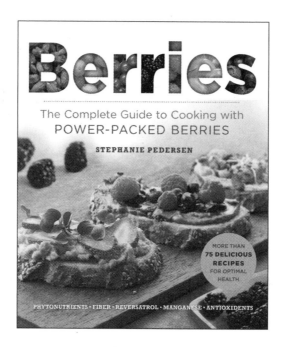

BERRIES

The Complete Guide to Cooking with Power-Packed Berries,
Stephanie Pedersen
978-1-4549-1835-6

Berries are outrageously delicious, convenient, and a potent health food that can help alleviate conditions as wide-ranging as heart disease, arthritis, diabetes, and cancer. Here, you'll find a complete guide to these superfoods with information on buying and storage, an overview of their nutritional benefits, and 75 tempting recipes for smoothies, appetizers, snacks, and meals—including decadent desserts and baked goods!